"Most diet books tell you wha[...]t [...]never [...]into the su[...] that really matters for sustained loss and change—the mindset—the reasons why we eat how we eat. *Peace with Food* goes into all of that WITHOUT telling you what to eat and still have success!"

~Siobhan Burch, Beachbody Coach

"As a former high school and collegiate wrestler, I know the frustration and the sea of negative emotions on the road to losing hundreds of pounds only to gain them back...plus more. I only wish this book were available years ago, because it provides many easy-to-use and practical tools that you can start using today to get permanent results. I highly encourage you to read this book now and choose the path that leads to: peace with food!"

~Bob Manard, Leadership and Speech Coach

"PWF (peace with food) is unlike anything I have tried before. For the first time in my life I am getting to know myself, I am trying new foods, and finally finding food enjoyable. This is the easiest, most fulfilling plan I have ever tried. It's not only helped me to make healthier food choices, I have found I am intentionally looking for peace in other areas of my life. I have stuck with this plan longer than anything I have tried in the past, and can say with confidence my life is richer in so many ways having found peace with food."

~Lisa Collins, Elementary Teacher

"Peace with food has filtered into other areas of my life. It really is that powerful."

~Wendy Taylor,
President and Founder of Freedom Trade International

PEACE

WITH

FOOD

Eat What You Want.
Never Diet Again.
Live a Happy Life.

Lara Shoup & Robynn Coates

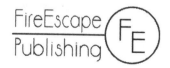

PEACEWITHFOOD
Eat What You Want. Never Diet Again. Live a Happy Life.

By Lara L. Shoup and Robynn K. Coates

ISBN-13: 978-0991164967
(FireEscape Publishing, LLC)

*Disclaimer: You have to be honest with yourself and be willing to face your struggles in order to benefit from this book. We hope this material serves as a guide in determining what measures are necessary to help you find peace with food. For some people it is following a plan, for others it will be a psychological issue that may require professional help.

We are not dietitians or physicians. Therefore, we don't endorse any specific eating plan. We will, however, share with you what has worked for us. Please visit with your physician to determine what kind of eating plan and exercise plan are right for you.

This book is dedicated to you.
May you finally be able to live at peace with food
and enjoy the best life ever.

"The secret to living well +
longer: eat half, walk double,
laugh triple, and love without
measure."
—Tibetan Proverb

Table of Contents

Acknowledgements

Wow, thank you to our husbands and kids. After years of weight fluctuation due to experimentation, early morning writing sessions, and endless conversations about our concepts, we can't thank you enough. You cut us a lot of slack on our roles as Mom, wife—you name it—all because you cheered us on to accomplish our dream of finishing this assignment. It is because of you that we can officially mark this endeavor as complete.

We are so grateful for everyone who helped us along the way. Thanks to our editors and those of you who dug through the trenches of proofing our book when it needed a lot of TLC. You know who you are—thank you for being open and honest in your feedback and for taking time out of your busy schedules to help. Your friendship means so much to us, and we are honored you could be part of the process.

And finally, to our favorite, God. Thanks for giving us the words, wisdom, and patience to write this book. None of this would have been possible without You.

Introduction

Happiness, not in another place, but this place…
not for another hour, but this hour.
~Walt Whitman

It was a typical hot summer night in Kansas. Our husbands were away supporting their alma mater's athletic program while we stayed with the kids at Robynn's house. As the sun went down, we sat on Adirondack chairs watching our little ones play in the backyard. Our conversation started like any other, but its ending was one we will never forget. That night while our kids caught fireflies in a mason jar, we captured lightning in a bottle.

Out of nowhere we were confessing our own secret struggles with eating. For the first time in our lives we let our guard down and spoke openly about weight, food, and self-image. The experience was unreal as we realized our crazy stories were so similar.

Capturing lightening in a bottle can be described as "catching something powerful." We caught something powerful that night— we learned we were not alone in our search for peace with food.

As the stars filled the dark sky, our honesty continued to lift an unimaginable weight. We admitted our embarrassing moments when it came to food…weak moments of going to the pantry and stuffing ourselves when no one was looking, times we'd compared ourselves to the models in a magazine. Our specific details may have been different, but our feelings and frustrations were the same.

For the next nine months we talked about this journey of finding peace. We discussed at length the struggles people face when it comes to their bodies and weight, and we considered the pressure our society and culture place on women in regard to this never-ending saga.

We decided not to rest until we found complete peace in these areas of our lives. We would not be satisfied until it became our new landscape, our new normal. So, with determination, we forged ahead.

How would we reach our objective? By being the scientists and conducting our own experiments. Fortunately, not only were we willing to try different methods to see which ones worked, but we also had years of failed weight loss attempts under our belts from which to draw valuable information. Because we had already tried countless diets and methods of losing weight, we didn't have many left to try.

And then after using the information we had gained from years of experimenting, it happened...

We caught a glimpse of the answer we had been searching for: peace with food.

We arrived at the same point, at the same time, even though the paths we took were quite different. Lara had been unsuccessfully trying to lose the last few pounds for almost a year and finally reached her breaking point. Robynn, on the other hand, had over twenty pounds to lose and had just tried the most restrictive diet she'd ever been on with no success. These experiences were the straw that broke the camel's back, causing us to draw a line in the sand, promising ourselves from that day forward we would never diet again.

In this book we detail the incredible one-eighty our lives have taken. You will see our painful struggles, specific strategies, and personal stories. When we say personal, that's exactly what this book is. You will step into our lives and see how we handle the food challenges life throws our way. Some of the stories will be our victories, but many will be examples of our failures and frustrations. We hope by sharing these, we'll help you experience the same freedom and peace we now have.

Other things we will discuss are:

- Why diets and rules don't work.
- How to overcome the subtle lie of our culture and society that says your value is based on your appearance.
- How to find out what you really want regarding your body and weight.

- How to deal with the all-or-nothing mindset that causes you to binge.
- How to handle uncomfortable, negative feelings and moods that lead to overeating.
- How to stop going to food for comfort.
- How to handle everyday situations, holidays, special occasions, and unexpected eating opportunities.
- How to create strategies with your body, weight, food, and exercise that will give you peace.
- How to get back on track at any moment instead of waiting until tomorrow, Monday, or January 1.
- How to deal with and successfully overcome temptation.

Our purpose in writing this book is simple: we want to share with others a revelation that has totally transformed our lives. This transformation includes how to live life on purpose, specifically in the area of eating. No more coasting along on auto-pilot, putting food in your mouth that you later regret. No more mindless eating that reaps dreadful results.

Let's get started!

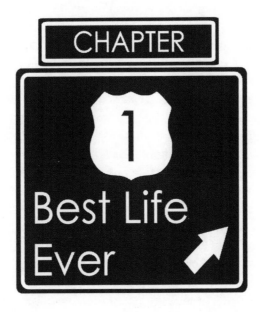

The Map

All you need is the plan, the road map, and
the courage to press on to your destination.
~Earl Nightingale

Luggage. Toll booth money. Car keys. These are all items you need
when taking a trip. But wait, don't forget an essential tool—your
map! That is exactly what this book will be for you as you take the
journey to peace with food. We call it *your* map because each
person is unique. The destination is the same—a life of peace—but
the trip to get there will vary with each driver. Therefore, no two
maps will be identical.

We know how exhausting traveling can be so we did you a
favor and gave you various rest stops along the way. These breaks

in your travel will provide a time of reflection—a time to evaluate your needs, both physical and psychological. While resting, you will answer questions to assist in setting a course specific to your own personal journey. This information is essential to finding the pathway tailored for none other than you. One designed to fit perfectly with your lifestyle, circumstances, preferences, and needs.

If you need examples to get started, we share our responses to the same questions under every rest stop. We hope you'll not only have the tools to figure out what paths to take, you also never have to worry about traveling alone. Road trips can be more fun as a group, so we are going to tag along as your Peace Coaches for added support. We will help you go through this, one step at a time. That is exactly what we did to get there. We made tiny positive choices on a daily basis, and as clichéd as it may sound, it has been life-changing.

When we started our own journey, we were open to whatever results we would uncover. We had no agenda or methods that answered our weight loss struggle. Instead, we were receptive to learning new lessons and making new discoveries. It was in this spirit of experimentation that we found the happiness we had desired for years.

In one of our all-time favorite family movies, *Tangled*, the lead character, Rapunzel, makes a statement we and our kids continue to repeat even years later: "Woo-hoo! Best. Day. Ever!" By living out this book, we too can say:

"Woo-hoo! This is the *Best. Life. Ever!*"

We truly feel this way, and life only gets better with each new vista.

We hope you'll come along.

It will be the *Best. Life. Ever!*

Meet Lara & Robynn

Life can only be understood backwards;
but it must be lived forwards.
~Soren Kierkegaard

Secret crushes. Best friends. High drama. These junior high moments are what we wrote about in our diaries back in the day. Reading them from time to time gives us a good laugh and reminds us of days gone by, a time when life was simple, opportunities were abundant, and we were young.

Although our writings today may have changed, we continue to put pen to paper. It's not because writing in a little diary complete with lock and key is the *in* thing to do. Instead we write to reflect. It helps us track our progress, look for trends, and reveal strengths and weaknesses.

In order for you to understand that we are ordinary and real people, just like you, we wanted to share our stories. Although our experiences and circumstances are unalike, one of the things we had in common was this: a secret struggle with food. Here are our diary entries:

Lara's Diary

Growing up, I didn't struggle with weight as much as I did self-image. I was a chubby kid in junior high, and after I hit a growth spurt in high school, staying thin didn't take much effort. Looking back though, I was never satisfied with my body. How sad when I look at pictures from back then.

It wasn't until I became pregnant with my first child that I was truly humbled with my weight. I gained over sixty pounds and looked so different, some people didn't even recognize me. I remember coming home from the hospital thinking, "This is it. I will no longer be able to wear skinny jeans." I believed it so much that I donated five trash bags of clothes to Goodwill within the first couple of months as a new mom.

Fast forward four years and another kiddo, and I wished I hadn't given up on myself so easily. I was able to eventually lose the weight and could have enjoyed some of those favorite outfits had I not given them away.

A couple of years after my second child, I was able to reach my lowest weight since 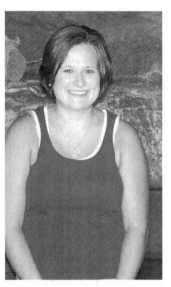 college. That was a huge accomplishment, but I continued to struggle with food and being happy with how I looked. I love sweets and had a hard time eating in moderation. One of my bad habits was sneaking food when no one was looking. I was guilty of opening a pantry door and hiding behind it while I threw food into my mouth. It was ugly, friends, let me tell ya. I even did this when my family was in the same room. It hurts to remember the struggle I had while doing this.

As if that isn't painful enough, whenever I let my guard down, I would end up eating thousands of calories more than my daily recommendation. This would result in discouragement for days, which would cause me to throw in the towel and continue to eat poorly for a week or so. Thankfully, I would eventually come to my senses and snap out of it. My life became a vicious cycle of giving in, porking out, feeling bad, having pep talks, then starting all over again by attempting to eat right and exercise. This happened repeatedly. That was my life. It was all I knew.

It wasn't until Robynn and I became close friends that I realized I wasn't alone. After we became determined to find an answer to this non-stop struggle, my life in many ways became instantly better. Sure, the experimental part was extremely challenging, but when you can finally take the reins and be in control of your life, there is something very freeing about that. I could see growth in this area with each step I took. That was so encouraging.

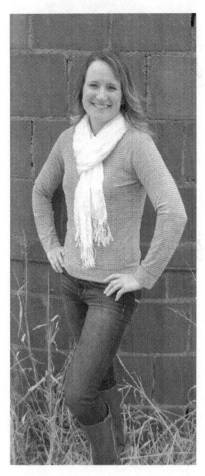

Now that I have peace with food, I still can't fully explain how I feel. At the very least, it's awesome! It's an amazing sense of freedom and control. And now that I have it, I can't imagine my life without it.

Robynn's Diary

It was during my sophomore year of high school that my weight and eating started to spiral out of control. A friend and I would frequently go to her grandma's house after school on the nights of ball games. On the

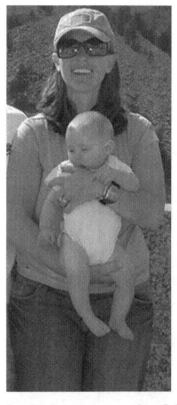

way there, we always stopped at the grocery store where we would buy a box of chocolate ice cream bars for snacks. I would finish off nine of the twelve while my friend would eat the other three. Needless to say, at the end of my sophomore year I had gained substantial weight.

During that summer I went on a diet and lost the weight and more. This began my infamous career of dieting. Although I could keep the unwanted weight at bay, it continually lurked over my shoulder. I remember one time being at home during my senior year of high school when a pan of toffee bars called my name from the kitchen. Although I didn't want to eat them, I can still hear the voice in my head saying, "You'll never be free." It was tormenting and I felt utterly defeated.

In college I gained the "Freshmen-15" plus some. My eating was so out of control. I can

honestly say I was addicted to food. I
thought about it constantly. Because it had
such a hold on my life, I went through
college overweight, defeated, and
discouraged. Food was my downfall, and I
couldn't get free.

During this time there were a couple of
individuals who spoke encouraging words into
my life regarding overcoming this addiction.
They told me I could be free. I held on to
that hope, and although I didn't experience
results immediately, their words were seeds
that were planted into my life. I am certain
the freedom I now have is due to what they
shared with me decades ago.

After college my life was a roller coaster
of diet, lose a little weight, and then gain
it all back. I had my doubts as to whether
or not I could even lose weight. But still,
I was determined. After the birth of my
second child, I decided I would go all out
and finally get down to the weight I desired
and where I felt the best at both physically
and emotionally. For about a year and a
half, I was on a hard core diet. I finally
lost all the weight I had wanted to lose and
more, but it required me to eat a strict
protein diet and exercise excessively.

At the end of my dieting stint, I lost all
control and gained all the weight back. Of
course, I tried to get back to strict
dieting to achieve the same results, but
something inside me resented this insanity
and refused to cooperate with another
restrictive diet.

It was shortly thereafter that Lara and I
had our *lightning in a bottle* conversation
on my back porch that would forever change

my life. Although it didn't happen all at once, step by step, I began to make changes in the way I thought about food, myself, and my body. And as my thoughts began to change, so did my life.

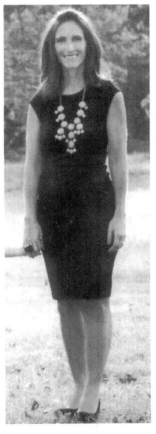

Dieting was replaced with healthy habits that I could live with for the rest of my life. Habits that would not only help me maintain my healthy weight, but would also allow me to enjoy my life and the people in it. And finally, my unhealthy get-thin-quick mindset was replaced with one that brought self-control, freedom, and happiness.

Experiencing this greater level of life was not something that occurred instantly. However, the moment I determined I would never diet again, I began experiencing it more than I had ever imagined, and it only gets better with every passing day. I can finally say that it's no longer the destination I'm focused on. Instead, I'm finally enjoying the journey.

If you can relate to our stories, have experienced the vicious cycle of diet, lose weight, gain weight, and then do it all over again, or you are at your goal weight but don't have peace, take heart. We can't begin to tell you how many people we've talked to who live in this frustrating state of existence. You are not alone.

The good news is you don't have to live like this. There is a better way. We'll soon be sharing the foundation of how to have peace with food, but for now, let's dive into the catalyst that started all this in the first place: our revelation that diets don't work.

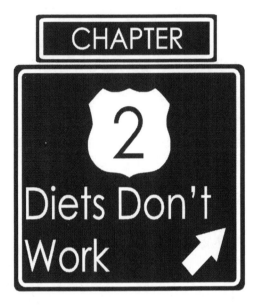

CHAPTER

2

Diets Don't Work

Missing Key Ingredients

Lara

Practically every day growing up, we came home from school to find my mom preparing homemade chocolate chip cookies. To this day, those are, hands down, my favorite cookie. Every time I eat one, it is accompanied by nostalgic thoughts of my childhood— seeing the reflection of my face as I looked through the glass oven door, watching each cookie rise while anticipating the first bite. I smell the sweetness as it makes its way through the house. Smiling, I pour a glass of milk, knowing that in a few minutes it will be shared with my favorite dessert.

The moment finally arrives. I sit down at the table and think how I've never seen a cookie that looked so good. I take the first bite…and…*Blech! Yuck!* "What happened?!" I scream as my mom runs in from the other room. Quickly she realized that baking powder was substituted for baking soda. Shucks! One wrong ingredient made all the difference in the outcome. The cookie looked perfect, but as soon as it hit my mouth, it made me cringe.

In the same way, diets are missing a few key ingredients needed to provide long-term success. In this chapter we'll be discussing why diets don't work.

Lacks a Permanent Solution

Doing more of what doesn't work won't make it work any better.
~ Charles J. Givens

Lara

Like most people, I decided to go on the exact same diet as someone I knew. This particular time it was my youngest sister. We stayed in close contact about what we were eating and how we were exercising, and we did our best to do everything the same. Before long, I experienced frustrations and couldn't help but share them with Robynn. I told her how my sister was losing weight and I was gaining, even though we were following the same diet plan. I mean, give me a break! I was following the same diet rules as someone from my own bloodline and still couldn't get the same results!

Let's face it, we are all unique from one another. What works for one may not work for another. Many people start a diet hoping it will be the answer to food obsession and out-of-control eating, but before long they are right back where they started.

Because the word *diet* means different things to different people, it is important that we give you our definition of a diet:

Diet = A temporary fix that lacks long-term peace.

Typically a diet* is an eating plan that consists of one or more of the following:

- Reduces your intake of food
- Restricts what you can eat

- Deprives you of foods you love
- Requires eating specific combinations of foods
- Tells you when you can eat
- Tells you what you can or cannot drink

And since we are talking about diets that don't work, it is also important that we give you our definition of the word *work*.

Work = A permanent solution that gives peace for life.

We agree that if you want to lose weight you will have to limit the amount of food you consume. That being said, we don't agree that you have to restrict yourself from eating your favorite foods, which we will discuss later in this book.

Diets don't work because they can't give you a permanent solution that can be achieved for life. To give you a better idea of what we mean, let's compare diets to going to the hair salon (so, gals, this one's for you). Imagine leaving the salon with the most beautiful hairstyle you've ever seen. You are *in love*. It is perfectly cut and has amazing volume, and the color shows no gray. Better yet, a follow-up appointment is unnecessary because your hair will never grow again and no upkeep is required. That would be awesome, to say the least!

> If you bought a car that worked only 60% of the time, it would be considered unacceptable. Why don't we look at diets the same way?

Unfortunately, we all know this scenario is unrealistic. And so are diets. But don't give up yet. There is something out there that works, and you are holding it in the palm of your hands: *Peace with Food*.

*If you are wondering about plans like Weight Watchers®, which are called diets, we would not consider them as one. The Weight Watchers® plan allows you to eat what you love, just not as much as you'd love to eat so you aren't deprived of foods you enjoy.

Too Much Focus on a Quick Fix

Imagine standing in a college auditorium dressed in cap and gown. You are handed your high-honors diploma, which states you now have a degree in engineering.

But hold on a second. There's one small catch. You didn't spend the five years learning the information. The diploma, with your name on it, was just given to you. You know absolutely nothing about engineering. And although the diploma lands you a high-paying job, you haven't considered how you are going to handle your first day of work, and every day after. Continuing in this job could be a disaster since you've had no training.

If we try to lose weight without learning how to maintain it later, it defeats the purpose. Sure, you may lose the weight, but if you gain it all back, it was a waste of time and energy. Keeping the pounds off won't be easy if your history consists of nothing but shortcuts to get there. Most people focus on losing the weight but never have a plan for when their goals are met.

Like getting a higher level education, it takes time. It takes patience. You have to go to class, take tests, and spend hours doing research. The same applies to peace with food. If you want maintaining your weight loss goal to be easy, put in the time now. You don't want to revert to the same restrictive diet after you gain the weight back, so consider investing your time into something that will last.

Diets don't work because they lack teaching on how to successfully maintain your weight, in peace, once you reach your goal. They put too much focus on a quick fix that will be troublesome when you lose the weight and then gain it all back. So say goodbye to those days. It's time we break this cycle, once and for all.

Results Are Not Typical

However beautiful the strategy, you should occasionally look at the results.
~Winston Churchill

If you look closely at the bottom of most diet ads you will quickly find the words *results not typical*. After being lured with photos of people who dropped twenty pounds in two weeks, we overlook these well-disguised, depressing facts. The truth is written right before us, yet we put more hope in the slim chance that we can obtain the same incredible weight loss results as they did.

We've all heard stories about the winners of million dollar lotteries. Days leading up to the drawing, people are frantically rushing to the convenience store purchasing as many tickets as they can. Maybe, just maybe, theirs will be the lucky number. Deep down everyone knows their chances of success are slim to none. It even crosses their minds that buying the ticket is a waste of money, but people buy them anyway in hopes of solving their financial problems.

We know how the story ends. Everyone, except one person, walks away feeling disappointed. Defeated. They wasted their paychecks on the lottery, yet continued to struggle to make car payments. The idea of quick cash from a possible winning sounded far more enticing than paying the bills. If only they had realized that working slowly and steadily at saving money would cause them less stress, not to mention, would have paid for their car outright.

People do this to themselves all the time. The obvious answer is right in front of them, yet they choose the quicker, bigger, faster approach. A person can't go on a strict diet for two months and expect to have the same, lasting results as the model in the advertisement. Ask these questions to evaluate yourself and those around you:

- How many diets have I tried?
- How long did they last?

- How many people do I know who stuck to a diet longer than a year?
- How many people do I know who lost weight on a diet, only to gain it right back when they went off the diet?

Research shows that when it comes to dieting, only a small percentage of people actually keep the weight off after five years. According to UCLA associate professor of psychology and researcher Traci Mann, although a person can initially lose five to ten percent of their weight on a diet, chances are they will regain the weight they originally lost. In her research on thirty-one different diets, Mann stated: "We found that the majority of people regained all the weight, plus more. Sustained weight loss was found only in a small minority of participants, while complete weight regain was found in the majority. Diets do not lead to sustained weight loss or health benefits for the majority of people."[1]

From our experience we can attest to these results: if you want a sure way to gain weight, go on a diet.

Diets don't work because they can't offer successful results to the majority of people. And many times, the long-term results are opposite of what they promise. You have the ability to stop putting yourself in a position of failing all of the time. The process may be slower, but peace with food can give you a lifetime of freedom.

Success Is Based on Inflated Weight

I have not failed. I've just found 10,000 ways that won't work.
~Thomas A. Edison

Robynn

Speaking of the fine print that reads, "Results Not Typical," you have probably seen the headlines, "Lose 10 Pounds in 10 Days," or something similar splashed across magazine covers.

Is it possible? Maybe. But consider this: How do people typically eat on the days leading up to a diet? Think of the times you went on a diet, say January first. Days prior, were you eating moderately? Or were you eating everything in sight?

Most likely you spent that time binging. You knew your favorite foods would be off-limits in the near future, so you took advantage of the last opportunity to feast.

We saw a series of posts on Facebook® by a group of people who were starting a restrictive diet the next day. Before they began, they planned a trip to a fast food restaurant for one final splurge. This is exactly what we are talking about. It is a perfect example of the diet mentality.

Because of this excessive feast, you don't begin your diet at what we call your baseline or set-point weight. When you begin a diet with a binge, your starting weight is most likely inflated eight to fifteen pounds, which, by the way, is typically the boast many diets say you can lose in two weeks.

Think about it. This is crazy! When you begin a diet with inflated weight, you can quickly lose eight to fifteen pounds on any diet that reduces your calories. I know, because I did just that while experimenting for this book. I went on what I call the Reese's® diet. After overeating and temporarily gaining weight, I ate only Reese's® Peanut Butter Cups, in moderation, for a few days. My result, not surprisingly, was losing those same eight to fifteen pounds, and I was back at my pre-feasting weight within days.

Diets don't work because they often base their success on inflated weight. So next time you are tempted to be wowed by the latest diet with audacious claims, remember it is no different from any other diet.

The Insane Cycle Dominates

Insanity: doing the same thing over and over again and expecting different results.
~Albert Einstein

It is crazy to think about all the insane actions we take to reach our goal weight: excessive workouts, strict diets, unrealistic rules, rigid plans, and deprivation. These are all things we have come to expect when starting a diet.

Throughout this book we will talk about the insane cycle. This is a concept we initially read about from the marriage book *Love and Respect* by Dr. Emerson Eggerichs (one we highly recommend, by the way). In *Love and Respect*, Dr. Eggerichs discusses how married couples get wrapped up in doing the same thing—over and over—in an unproductive, destructive manner. He calls this the "crazy cycle." A similar cycle exists in seeking peace with food. We call this our insane cycle.

The following were some of our antics of repetitive insanity before we wrote this book. Do any of these sound familiar?

- Thinking the only way to get back on track is to not eat for a few days.
- Feeling like a failure when unexpected events caused us to overeat.
- Stepping on the scale multiple times a day.
- Thinking that food would satisfy when we were in a funk or having a bad day.
- Not realizing our obsession with weight was stealing our enjoyment and quality of life.
- Allowing little slip-ups to turn into full-fledged mess-ups.
- Buying healthy foods we didn't like but felt obligated to get, only to pitch them weeks later because they spoiled in the fridge.

Speaking of the insane cycle, it reminded Robynn of a time she was so focused on the number of her ultimate weight goal, she couldn't enjoy being the lowest weight she'd ever been, even though she felt and looked great. Lara recalled when she and a friend were so obsessed with being the same skinny size, they measured every part of their body and compared results. Lara would also weigh in after working out and, if she showed even a one-pound gain, she would go eat until she was stuffed, convinced exercising wasn't working, so why bother?

Diets don't work because they contribute to the continuation of the insane cycle, causing you to make questionable choices and not think clearly. The insane cycle doesn't take us where we want to be. Instead, it always takes us right back where we started. Peace with food will not only end this never-ending cycle, but it will give you a level of happiness you never thought possible.

The Blame Is Put on Food

If you take responsibility for yourself you will develop a hunger to accomplish your dreams.
~Les Brown

Diets do not lead to sustained weight loss or health benefits for the majority of people, yet we continue this madness. We carry on with the insanity of doing the same thing over and over, expecting different results, because there doesn't seem to be any other option besides dieting.

In our quest for a healthy lifestyle, we discovered that being allowed to enjoy foods that diets said were bad actually brought a great deal of peace. By eating these foods in a controlled manner, we gained enjoyment, an improved quality of life, and a greater level of self-control.

You might think giving yourself permission to enjoy favorite foods, whether they be classified as healthy or unhealthy, would give you a license to indulge and cause your eating to spiral out of control. Surprisingly, the opposite was true for us. When we gave ourselves permission to eat what we wanted, as long as it gave peace, we naturally began to eat healthier. It took time, but we found allowing forbidden food actually diminished the pull of food. This experiment proved food was not the problem—yet another difference from diets.

Diets don't work because they play the blame game. They make food the problem. In some diets the problem is carbohydrates, in others it is foods high in fat. We were surprised to see in some diets that even fruits and vegetables were considered to be problematic.

We don't subscribe to this belief. Rather than placing the blame on certain foods, we believe the responsibility lies within us. It is our mismanagement of food, lack of skill, lack of knowledge or a combination of all these, that results in an unhealthy and overweight body.

If there are foods the body does react to negatively, such as gluten to the person with celiac disease or carbs to the diabetic, the eating problems are not completely resolved once these culprits are eliminated. This person still needs to exercise self-control and moderation if she or he wants to be healthy.

As you read through this book, you will come across one of our mantras:

You can eat whatever you want, as long as it brings you peace.*

We realize this is a bold statement. To the dieter, it may even seem blasphemous. But as you begin to walk in peace with food, you will discover that your approach to food will change. It may result in learning to eat your favorite unhealthy foods in moderation. Or maybe it will mean removing foods from the pantry that repeatedly cause you to overeat. Regardless, the bottom line is this: You are responsible for your life. It is not the responsibility of the food, the diet, or another person. The responsibility lies solely with you.

If you are feeling discouraged because you are well aware you've been the one responsible for your life, but feel you've let yourself down thus far, take heart. You can't change what you don't know. This book will give you all the tools to help you have a relationship with food in a new and improved way. Once you finish reading, you'll know better, which will help you do better from here on out. So hang tight. Don't be so hard on yourself. There is more yet to learn.

*For the majority of people, this principle applies. However, because there is no one-size-fits-all, you may have to adjust this according to your specific needs. This would include, but is not limited to, those who are diabetic or have celiac disease or some other issue requiring strict monitoring of food intake.

Heavily Influenced by *They*

Back in the 1950s and early 60s, Marilyn Monroe was an icon. Beautiful, curvy and voluptuous. In her day, that was *in* and looking anorexic was not so *in*. However, if the young Marilyn were living today, she would no doubt be on the latest and greatest diet promising instant success to fulfill *their* ridiculous standards. Notice how we treat *They*. Like *They* are some supreme being with ultimate knowledge about how we should conduct our lives:

- *They* say you shouldn't wear…
- *They* say you can't eat…
- *They* say you must exercise…

No one really knows this infamous entity called *They,* yet we give them authority over our lives, and the power *They* wield is phenomenal. *They* tell us how to dress and how to raise our kids. Invariably, what *They* deem acceptable today becomes outdated tomorrow.

Diets don't work because *They* don't even know us and our unique circumstances. The crazy thing is, we still let them tell us what to do and expect successful results! If you are tired of abiding by a set of rules imposed by an anonymous group of people, it is time to kick *They* to the curb. Start living a life in which you make all the calls.

It's a One-Size-Fits-All Approach

Imagine you are sick and you make an appointment to see a doctor. You enter the clinic, check in, and to your surprise, the receptionist hands you a prescription without even conferring with the doctor. She tells you to fill the prescription and follow the instructions. She guarantees that doing so will alleviate your problem.

Stunned, you notice everyone around you is holding the same prescription. All patients are given one diagnosis and one set of instructions.

This one-size-fits-all scenario probably sounds familiar to you when it comes to diet plans, but don't discredit creating a lifestyle that is tailored specifically for you. We don't believe a single eating plan is the answer. We are complex people with a plethora of factors that must be considered.

Diets don't work because they are a one-size-fits-all approach. No two people are the same. Each person has her or his own set of unique circumstances. For example, take a look at the differences between the two of us:

Exercise
Lara: I run a home-based business in addition to taking care of my kids. Although I struggle to find time for traditional exercise, I spend most of the day on my feet. By staying active around the house, I can burn the calories needed to offset what I eat.

Robynn: I enjoy a variety of ways to exercise. I may run, walk, or do strength training, depending on my mood. My schedule allows time for daily exercise, which is something I enjoy.

Must Haves
Lara: I insist on having a dessert at night. I savor this time of day because I can finally sit down and relax after all my kids are snug in their beds.

Robynn: I savor eating early in the morning, before the kids wake up. This is "my" time.

Food
Lara: I love veggies and protein. Everyone in my family is a huge fan of protein and having meat in every meal is a must!

Robynn: I don't love veggies (unless they are fresh from the garden) and don't miss protein if it isn't on the table. With both veggies and protein, I have to intentionally plan them in my meals.

When it comes to food and exercise, one can see how different we are. We can both accomplish the same goal but take different paths to get there.

It's a Lab Setting, Not the Real World

Don't be afraid to challenge the pros, even in their own backyard.
~Colin Powell

Scary. That's what becoming your own scientist can be. In our fast-paced society we are accustomed to vast quantities of information coming at us at breakneck speeds. It's hard to know what is relevant and what is obsolete. When to hit "Delete" and when to hit "Save."

As a result, you let others do the thinking for you. But remember, *They* don't know you. *They* conduct research in controlled settings and give you their results suggesting you follow their rules. But you don't live in a lab setting. You live in the real world—a place with ever-changing circumstances that may defy their rules.

You have to take authority over your life. Even someone who knows you well (spouse, sibling, best friend) can't make decisions for your life as well as you can. You are the only one who lives, breathes, and thinks the way you do. This is why you need to have the final say and decide what's best for your situation.

Peace with food allows you to be in control. It allows you to maneuver through the tricky moments life deals you and emerge with flying colors. Diets and rules can't do that. They don't work because they are rigid and don't take into account the everyday eating situations life presents.

We aren't discrediting the results science may find. In fact, we encourage you to find out what research is saying. But we also understand that there is a plethora of information on dieting, health, and fitness, and deciding which advice you should follow can leave you downright confused. There is no need to worry because we will help you gain victory in your life by teaching you how to seek out wisdom and get knowledge on your specific situation. You will gain confidence in learning how to sift through the diet and health information and use what will fit within your unique lifestyle.

Here is another piece of advice: Get information from someone who does not have a dog in the fight. By all means, read about different strategies for health or fitness in order to find techniques you may like, but also inform yourself with research from unbiased, reputable, scientific sources. The following individuals should have your best interest in mind:

- Certified dietitians who can help advise you how to eat nutritiously and reach health-related goals.
- Doctors who can give an overall assessment of your health. If you don't feel like your doctor is the right fit, shop around and find one who suits you best.
- Scientific researchers who have no incentive to report results one way or the other.
- Local university extension offices who can help interpret nutrition research.

So as you are approached by new weight loss information, ask yourself if each eating plan will work for you. Consider whether it will give peace, whether it is nutritionally balanced, whether it promotes your health and well-being, and whether it is something you can do for life. Your answers will probably vary, which is what this process is all about: learning how to take what you know and create a successful lifestyle that is tailor made specifically for you.

Speaking of which, let's take a moment at our first rest stop to reflect on some ideas. Jot down key characteristics regarding your unique life that diets overlooked. Why have diets failed you in the past? What should they know about *you*?

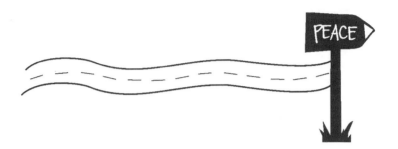

A. The Bookstore

Your Story—What are your personal situations, circumstances, and idiosyncrasies in your life that diets didn't take into consideration, causing you to fail?

- _____
- _____
- _____
- _____
- _____

Lara: I have to plan ahead with groceries because I live in the country and only go to the grocery store once a week. I also love to eat at night when the kids are in bed, the house is quiet, and I can watch my favorite television show. I save my sweet tooth for this time of day because I know I will be able to savor it the most during that time.

Robynn: Injuries requiring me to walk rather than run. I have kids who aren't old enough to be home alone, so I have to either work out in the morning or get a grandparent to watch my kids. I love eating in the car on road trips. It doesn't happen often, but when it does, it is comfort food for me. I also like to eat early in the morning when it is still quiet in the house.

Chapter 2 Take-Home Messages

Diets don't work because:

✓They can't give you a permanent solution that gives peace for life.

✓They lack teaching on how to successfully maintain your weight in peace once you reach your goal.

✓They can't offer successful results to the majority of people.

✓They might base their success on inflated weight.

✓They contribute to the continuation of the insane cycle, causing you to make questionable choices and not think clearly.

✓They play the blame game by making food the problem.

✓They don't know you and your unique circumstances.

✓They are a one-size-fits-all approach.

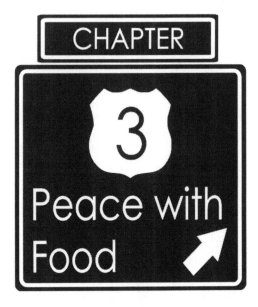

CHAPTER

3

Peace with Food

What Is Peace with Food?

Robynn

Ahhh…the coveted Super Bowl ring. It's big, it's flashy, and it's the dream of countless men (and boys) wishing they could earn the title that would secure such a prize. For a few fortunate, one isn't enough. They may have two—or three. But for most, just having one would be a dream come true. Once you win that title, it's for life. No one can take it away, request a rematch, or challenge you to another contest. From that point on you will forever be a Super Bowl champ.

Unfortunately, we have some good news and we have some bad news. The bad news is there is no Super Bowl ring when it comes to peace with food. Because, let's face it, this is a forever journey. There are no quick fixes and you are going to have to enlist for life.

For the long haul. It will never be something you can officially mark off your to-do list.

Now for the good news: peace with food is not only possible, it is worth fighting for. It will revolutionize your existence. You can experience the freedom of not being obsessed with thoughts of food and it will give you a new lease on your future. Best of all, you can begin having it today.

All my life I had a love-hate relationship with food. Love and hate, but never peace. Food had always been there to temporarily relieve me of stress when I had a bad day. It was there to make me feel deprived when I was trying to lose a few pounds. It made me miserable after I pigged out. My life was all those things, but definitely not peace.

When was the last time you went on a diet that talked about having happiness and freedom with food? Or how about a diet that promised—and delivered—lasting results? What a concept!

All of this may be a new idea for you, something you have never considered possible until now. But it *is* a possibility. It can become your new landscape, the new way you live. Trust us when we say it is possible. We are flat out telling you that you can succeed at this!

Peace with food will look different for each person, but here are some basic similarities:

- Having a clear mind instead of being obsessed with and fixated on food.
- Controlling your eating vs. having a diet control you.
- Feeling satisfied with foods you eat vs. feeling deprived.
- Having freedom in your eating. Eating what you want vs. thinking you must stick to a rigid plan.
- Giving yourself permission to enjoy the food you desire when hungry; you stop eating when you are satisfied, but not full.
- Eating something you want, in a controlled manner. As a result, a switch has been turned off in your mind, and you no longer think about food.
- Moving food or dieting from the center of your life to its proper place.

We hope such a prospect is enticing to you, because it has totally transformed our lives. It has set us free when it comes to food and diets. Let's dive in as we continue answering the question, "What exactly is peace with food?"

Follow and Rate Your Peace

Every human being must have boundaries in order to have successful relationships or a successful performance in life.
~Henry Cloud

If we were to sum up this book in a short phrase it would be this:

Follow peace.

But if you're new to pursuing peace, that may be too abstract. What does it look like? What does it feel like?

Imagine a picturesque pasture with rolling green hills and a beautiful blue sky with white puffy clouds. Surrounding the pasture is a fence enclosing the usual black-and-white cows grazing on the luscious green grass. Maybe the picture is from Wisconsin, maybe California, but regardless it beckons you to come stay a while. The scene is serene and inviting. A place you would like to visit and maybe even linger for some time. This is a picture of peace with food. It is like a green pasture surrounded by a fence—a boundary. A boundary that very clearly distinguishes what is in and what is out.

In your quest for this new way of life, it is imperative you find your green pasture. In the upcoming diagram, we've included a *Peace Chart* to help pinpoint the different levels you may experience. At first it may be challenging to determine where you fall on the chart, however, you will find that as you continue to practice, you will eventually master this skill.

We were thrilled to find this chart doesn't just work in the area of food, exercise, and your body, but in other areas of life as well. For example, when Lara becomes overwhelmed with her schedule, she lists her commitments and utilizes the chart to determine what activities are lacking peace. This helps her decide what activities need adjustments or need to be declined in the future.

Peace with food helps track your progress by rating your actions and decisions. As soon as you sense a lack of control, you can make necessary adjustments to get back on track. Always remember: when in doubt, follow peace.

Your green pasture awaits.

RATE YOUR PEACE
What's your level of peace?

 5 Peace!!
"I've got this!"
Happy, Free & In Control

 4 Mostly Peace
"Can't complain. Feeling Good!"
Satisfied, Content

 3 Some Peace
"Ok."
Mild Deprivation

 2 A Little Bit of Peace
"Could be worse, but I've seen better days."
Feeling a little cruddy

 1 Very Little Peace
"Help! I feel like I'm about to spiral out of control!"
Frustrated & Lack of Control

 0 No Peace At All
"I'm Hopeless."
Sad, Complete Lack of Control,
Beyond Discouraged

Build Your Character

Character cannot be developed in ease and quiet. Only through experience of trial and suffering can the soul be strengthened, ambition inspired, and success achieved.
~Helen Keller

When you think of the word *peace*, what comes to mind? Maybe it is the feeling you get after the kids are in bed, the house is quiet, and you can finally sit back and relax. Perhaps it is best depicted when you are taking a walk or listening to your favorite song. Whatever it may be, it is something we all enjoy and want more of.

We define peace with food as a state of tranquility—a place where you can be satisfied with yourself and with food. It is not being fixated on food but being fully engaged in life.

Peace with food helps build character. In fact, we say it is an inside job. That is one reason we don't promise lightning-speed results. Character isn't developed in two weeks or five days or in time for swimsuit season (or whatever promise the latest and greatest diet is making).

Not being able to lose excess pounds or lacking happiness are not external, superficial issues, but rather, they constitute an inside job. There are certain character traits you will learn through your journey, but the cool thing is, they will benefit you in all aspects of life. Let's take a look:

- **Patience**—Being able to calmly stick to the task, which leads us to…
- **Endurance and Perseverance**—Going through the uncomfortable stages and continuing on, even when the going gets rough and takes longer than anticipated.
- **Self-Control**—Being able to adjust your behavior despite what your feelings or circumstances tell you.
- **Peacefulness**—The ability to:
  - Accept what you cannot change and move on.
  - Change what is in your realm of responsibility.
  - Enjoy the entire process no matter where you are.

- **Attentiveness and Wisdom**—Being conscious and doing things on purpose rather than living on auto-pilot.
- **Inventiveness**—Developing the skill to aptly maneuver through tempting and challenging moments.
- **Optimism**—Being proactive and positive.
- **Kindness**—Giving yourself grace rather than expecting perfectionism.
- **Adaptability**—flexible rather than rigid.
- **Decisiveness**—Being a master game planner and strategist rather than indecisive and vague.

Now don't panic. If you struggle with any of these character traits that doesn't mean you are doomed to fail. This process is unique. It allows you to improve upon these areas of character (which will benefit other areas of your life as well) while still making progress with your weight loss goal.

There's a quote attributed to Chinese philosopher and poet Lao Tzu that says:

> **Watch your thoughts, for they become words.**
> **Watch your words, for they become actions.**
> **Watch your actions, for they become habits.**
> **Watch your habits, for they become character.**
> **Watch your character, for it becomes your destiny.**

These characteristics go way beyond your relationship with food and are transferable to the rest of your life. So, although it may take a little time before you begin to see progress, keep making the right choices. They are determining your destiny.

Robynn: For me, peace with food came *before* arriving at my desired goal weight. That's right, before! I'll admit, I wasn't thrilled about it. My thoughts were, "Let me get to my goal weight and then I will spend forever working on the inside stuff. Just get me to my goal weight!" Can you see my lack of patience and self-control? Thankfully that

prayer wasn't answered and instead I had to
learn to do things the right way before
seeing results.

Simplify Your Life

A little simplification would be the first step toward rational living, I think.
~Eleanor Roosevelt

We have all heard the phrase, "Simplify your life." If you were to simplify your busy schedule, you would start by prioritizing your commitments and eliminating activities that take up too much of your time. If you were a college student preparing for finals, you would simplify your studying by writing key points on note cards versus flipping through hundreds of pages in the book.

Peace with food is exactly what the word *simplify* is all about. When you don't simplify, stress occurs. See if any of this sounds familiar:

> We stress about our weight, so we go on a crazy diet. The diet makes us hungry, which causes us to be cranky. When the diet doesn't give the results we want, we increase our time at the gym, which means giving up even *more* family time. When your daughter's birthday party arrives, you pass up eating cake because you are still trying to diet. Not eating the cake makes you feel deprived. Later that night, after everyone is asleep, you step on the scale to see if your lack of eating has helped you lose weight. Nope. A one pound gain! So what do you do? Sneak out and gorge yourself with leftover cake. This is your attempt to make up for all the ways your diet and exercise deprived and failed you.

Does this situation sound familiar? One could quickly diagnose this as the insane cycle. To stop the madness, we can prescribe the act of simplifying. So let's try this again. If you simplify that same scenario, it would sound more like this:

You don't stress about your weight or go on crazy diets because you can eat what you want, as long as it gives peace. You know the weight will naturally drop as long as you stay focused on your journey. You aren't starving, which keeps you from being cranky. This improves your relationships because you aren't on edge all the time. You exercise, but in a way that works best for your schedule and brings you happiness. You always take the stairs and walk during lunch so you can head home after work to spend time with your family. You get to eat the cake at your daughter's birthday party and be present for every special moment because you aren't controlled by food. And when midnight rolls around, you will be sound asleep because you wouldn't think twice about weighing yourself at a time that is not optimal.

If you have experienced simplifying areas in your life, you know how calming it is to think of the results. That is how we can best describe peace with food. Like all things in life, there will be occasional road blocks, but even with those, you can learn how to make adjustments to get your life back on track for continued tranquility.

Eliminate Deprivation

Robynn

Have you ever finished a diet through which you got down to your goal weight, looked and felt great, only to take a nose dive and start a free fall you can't stop? When you finally hit bottom, the results are disastrous. The weight you lost is back (and more), and your self-confidence has plummeted.

This phenomenon is commonplace and predictable when it comes to dieting. We have experienced it too many times to count.

With all the success and confidence you feel when nearing your goal weight, you seem to be soaring. Your deprivation and extreme sacrifice has paid off. Or so you think.

But there is a law at play here. It is Newton's Third Law of Motion, which says, "For every action there is an equal and opposite reaction."

This takes me back to my schoolteacher days where I taught students this law in science. I never thought for a moment I would teach this outside of class, but it happens to be very applicable to every area of your life.

You can easily understand this law by visualizing a pendulum. If you pull back the resting pendulum as high as you can and then release it, it will swing just as high in the opposite direction. If you pull back the pendulum just slightly, the pendulum will swing in the opposite direction to the same slight elevation.

The same is true in how you eat and diet. When you place excessive restrictions on how or what you eat and deny yourself the opportunities to eat in enjoyable settings, it's like pulling the pendulum back to its maximum height. Eventually, when let go, the pendulum will swing to its maximum elevation in the opposite direction. This causes you to binge and spiral out of control.

Lara and I have seen beauty pageants in which contestants were asked what they would do once the pageant was over. On one occasion, a contestant said she would eat Kentucky Fried Chicken. On another, the host handed out donuts to the eliminated contestants because they could finally eat carbohydrates. It's obvious these gals were craving what they had been deprived of. It would be interesting to know whether it caused them to lose control with food for the weeks and months following their pageant.

My husband, Scott, experienced this same phenomenon every year in high school. As a wrestler, he would have to diet each wrestling season. He remembers depriving himself during Thanksgiving when everyone else was eating all his favorite foods. And when wrestling season was over, he and his wrestling buddies would indulge for months.

Scott never had an issue with food and doesn't to this day, but even so, the extreme deprivation took its toll. He would eventually get back to normal eating and by summer would have lost the extra weight gained in the few months of overeating after wrestling season.

So, if this law of motion is in play even for the person who has no issue with food, why do you think it won't affect you when you go on a restrictive and extreme diet?

Peace with food stops the feelings of deprivation. In return, it eliminates the spiraling-out-of-control behavior that causes you to binge. It's time to gain control of that pendulum and put an end to the consequences of deprivation.

Experiment to Find What Works

All truths are easy to understand once they are discovered. The point is to discover them. That takes investigation.
~Galileo

There it was, on the checkout aisle. In quotes: "Lose three inches in three days!" Every time you go to the store, no doubt there will be a new diet on the front cover of one or more magazines, each promising instant results. It can be overwhelming deciding which one to choose. Should you pick the one that cuts carbs and is high in protein? How about the thirteen-day plan where you drink a gallon of water each day and eat celery at the prescribed times? Okay, we are being a bit facetious here, but it really isn't much different from some of the rigid plans out there.

Then there's the well-known rules to lose weight:

- Never eat in the car.
- Eat breakfast like a king, lunch like a prince, and dinner like a pauper.
- Never eat after 6 p.m.
- Don't eat fruit or carbs after 2 p.m.
- Eliminate certain foods altogether.
- Eat specific combinations of certain foods.

What's even more confusing is when certain foods are allowed on one diet but eliminated altogether on another. So, regardless what plan you pick, you feel like a failure.

The downside to all of these rigid plans is that they don't consider your individual circumstances, needs, and preferences.

Some people have health conditions that don't allow certain foods to be eaten. Others may have an eating schedule that isn't aligned with what the diet prescribes.

When we were growing up, both of our fathers were farmers. For Lara, dinnertime wasn't until the sun went down, which meant her family ate at 9 p.m. Robynn's family didn't eat as late, but many evenings it was after 7 p.m. Gathering around the table was when the family connected after working a long, hard day. Not to mention, these meals were usually the biggest of the day, including meat and potatoes, and ending with dessert.

We are not saying you should use every possible excuse to have poor eating habits. You must be realistic and decide what you can sacrifice and what is sacred. If eating a meal with your family is your most valued time of day, you probably don't want to omit that experience. Look at your life and decide what will fit best. Consider all factors in the equation.

Another option is to make modifications so you can still enjoy that awaited family time. If you don't want to eat late in the day, you could participate by drinking a cup of coffee or eating a salad or small portion of what the family is eating. Whatever you do, if it is a cherished time of your day and brings you peace, don't miss out on the experience merely because it is breaking a food rule.

A diet book that tells you what to do doesn't mean their prescribed method will work for you and your lifestyle. Instead, be your own scientist. Peace with food is about giving yourself the authority to come up with what works best for your situation. So let's discover what your needs are so you can gain complete control over your life, once and for all.

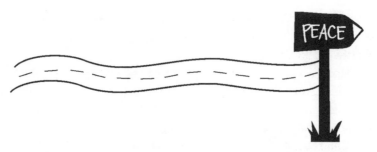

B. The Lab

Be the Scientist— What diet "rules" have you adapted to fit your lifestyle because they have proven to be successful for you?

- _____
- _____
- _____
- _____
- _____
- _____
- _____

Lara: It is suggested that eating more often during the day will make you less likely to overeat at meal times. After hearing this, I tried it out and have to agree. I eat less at dinner when I allow myself to have snacks during the day. This doesn't mean I only eat fruits and vegetables. I try to eat food that will fuel my body, but also food that I enjoy. For example, I often have an apple with peanut butter or trail mix with chocolate chips. If it keeps me from overeating during main meals, a slight indulgence with my healthy snack is actually a good thing.

Robynn: "Don't drink your calories." I totally agree with that. And the other diet rule I abide by is not eating at night.

Find What Keeps You in the Game

Lara

Anyone can relate to the time of year when people start panicking about losing weight before they hit the beach or attend their class reunion. What works best for you to kick those last few pounds? It may be going through the pantry and throwing out all of the junk food, giving up chocolate, or running a mile a day.

For me it is wearing clothing that makes me feel skinny. When I wear my skinny clothes, I eat better. If I wear an oversized t-shirt and mesh shorts, I might as well be holding a bag of Oreos, because that is what I will turn to after I look in the mirror! To be honest, at times I only had one or two outfits that made me feel really good. Since I was limited on these outfits, I only wore them in the evenings (when I struggled the most with eating). Better yet, when these clothing items became limited, it meant a shopping trip was in order. *Wink.*

I realize my answer may be different from yours. Just remember, every person is unique, so it is important to figure out what will keep you in the game. What is going to help you stay the course of following peace? Don't get frustrated if you are trying to follow the same plan as your co-worker or friend and the results are different. If giving up sweets—like they are—causes you to overcompensate later, then agree to eat (and enjoy) one or two cookies every day.

If you hate working out, then do something else. Your front yard has been begging for a facelift, and being outdoors always lifts your spirits, so consider redoing the landscaping in your flowerbeds. You can burn calories and, better yet, get an item marked off your to-do list.

Peace with food encourages finding what will keep you in the game. Discovering this will help increase your happiness, and as a result, your goals will be more attainable.

Choose the Outcome of Your Life

Look for your choices, pick the best one, then go with it.
~Pat Riley

We are going to make a very bold statement, one you may have a hard time believing. But it is true nonetheless. And that statement is:

You are powerful.

We're not talking about powerful in an invincible sort of way or powerful in a controlling kind of way. Rather, we are talking about powerful in the sense that you can determine whether your life will be productive and fulfilling or meaningless and unfulfilling. This choice lies in your hands completely.

With every situation you face, you have choices. Many times, you won't necessarily be pleased with all of the options, but the bottom line remains the same: you have choices. If you live in America or any other privileged country, you most likely have the latest

> You can stay where you are or you can choose a better path.

technology, conveniences, comforts, and opportunities available. But even if you don't, you still have the power of choice.

We read heroic stories of people who refused to complain or feel sorry for themselves, even in hellish conditions. Instead they chose a higher path. They looked at the opportunities rather than the terrible conditions, and as a result, lived a life of purpose, contentment, and even of power.

Take a good look at your life. Do you like what you see? If not, what are you doing to correct those things? Maybe you are forty pounds overweight and have been most of your adult life. Maybe you are on the brink of financial disaster or have crumbling relationships. If so, what are you doing about it?

Peace with food gives you the power to make a choice. Even if your situation is beyond your control, you get to choose whether you will spend your time complaining or being grateful for what you have and working toward a better future.

And what about those good intentions to make a choice? Those good intentions you never get around to? Well, the failure to choose is actually a choice in itself to stay right where you are.

If you need a little push out of the nest, we will be here to help you fly. We will help you make a choice to live the life that was intended for you. All it takes is a choice.

Fly, little birdie, fly.

Live Intentionally

The future starts today, not tomorrow.
~Pope John Paul II

It was story time at the local library. That is where our friendship began. It all started when Robynn came up to Lara and introduced herself. We spoke of things that many acquaintances would: our hobbies, kids, life, etc…

Fast forward two years. Our friendship had grown, and although it was more than surface level, not once had we shared our secret struggle with food.

Whether it was dieting, weight gain, feeling controlled by food, or uncertainty about what to eat, for years we both experienced the same vicious cycle.

Although the degree to which we struggled was different, we shared the same battle. We certainly were not living a life free of this distraction and we were tired of this scenario. We knew there had to be a better way. Bottom line, we wanted to be intentional: Live each day to the fullest, not obsessed with food, our bodies, or our weight. We wanted to savor life with all its highs, lows, and everything in-between.

Living in the moment and being satisfied with your present situation can be difficult, especially if your goals seem out of reach. Gaining contentment will finally allow you to make the best of your circumstances. With this mindset you can at last enjoy your current place in life even if it's not where you want to stay.

How can you be more intentional? For us, it is buying clothes that fit and flatter at our current weight and joining our kids at the pool. We don't want to postpone fun activities until we reach our goal weight. We want to cherish the moments around us and get excited about what the future holds. After all, looking perfect in a bathing suit isn't what's most important. Reaching your goal will come, but there is no reason to put your life on pause in the meantime.

These insignificant factors are controlling your life and stealing precious, limited time with those dearest to you. This journey is about embracing the present moment. Start investing in what matters most and live more intentionally today!

Benefit from a Posse

So we've talked about following and rating your peace, finding what keeps you in the game, building your character, and embracing life. You are very capable of doing all of these things on your own because this book includes the tools to help you do so. But there is something that will make your journey even better. Take it with a friend.

Sharing your experiences with someone else has many advantages. They can see things more accurately and have an unbiased perspective. They can offer support and be a listening ear with your decision making. This is what the two of us constantly do: bounce things off of each other and get each other's take on the situation. When we do, our view is always clearer.

If you've ever seen a good ol' western movie, you are probably familiar with the scene of cowboys appearing through a cloud of dust as they ride into town on horseback. They are decked out in cowboy hats, chaps, and boots, and are armed with a gun, ready to work together as they take on any criminal that dares to break the law. This group of men, more commonly referred to as a *Posse*, shared a common purpose by helping the sheriff keep the community free from harm.

We felt like these cowboys were onto something. We liked the idea of rallying together with friends and supporters, just like the westerners did with their posse. Except instead of working to enforce the law, your posse will be a significant component in your success. In fact, we believe in it so much that we created a *Posse Discussion Guide* in the back of this book to assist you along this journey.

Peace with food thrives most when utilizing the support of others. Finding the right posse will be important because you need to be surrounded with trustworthy individuals who have your best interests in mind. If finding a group seems impossible at this time, then find one other person, a Posse Partner, which can be just as beneficial.

Business as Usual

Take the first step in faith. You don't have to see the whole staircase, just take the first step.
~Martin Luther King, Jr.

Robynn
What an amazing feeling it was to see my all-time low on the scale on July 4, 2009, and then seven pounds lower less than a year later. As incredible as those all-time lows felt, they were short-lived. And when I say short-lived, I mean less than twelve hours, because once I hit my new low, something inside me panicked. All I wanted to do was eat my favorite food because I had been depriving myself and working out feverishly. I even had a long list of all the foods I would eat once my diet was over!

This all changes when you choose to walk in peace with food from the get-go, because you get to enjoy the foods you love and learn how to stay inbounds. This is also the secret to maintenance.

Maintenance is simply *business as usual*. The same steps that got you there will keep you there. The only thing you may need to change is adding a few extra calories so you don't continue to lose weight. How awesome is it that the lifestyle allowing you to lose weight with joy is also the answer to successful maintenance for life?

So as you are laying the groundwork for your journey, you are acquiring all the skills you will need for maintenance. It may take time, but it's worth it.

This doesn't mean you won't have challenges or experience the occasional funk. Eating in a way that gives peace won't *always* be easy. Over time you will acquire the skills and the wisdom you need. It's as if the medicine will be in the cabinet and will be yours for the taking. No gimmicks, no new plans, just business as usual.

Experience the Freedom of Peace

Lara

Every New Year's Eve looked the same. It was the unchanged story of the insane cycle. I ate all my favorite foods until the drop of the ball at midnight. I remember in high school when I ate puppy chow—that irresistible combination of Chex cereal covered in peanut butter, chocolate, and powdered sugar—and was completely stuffed when the clock struck midnight.

The image continues to be vivid in my mind: after I left the party, I sat in my car being tormented by the container in which handfuls of that yummy concoction remained. "But no more," I reminded myself. It was 12:18 a.m. and I had sworn to myself I would finally make a change and stick to a diet this time. Nevertheless, as with any insane cycle, you know how the story ends. The similar feelings were back to haunt me within months or even days because, once again, my overly ambitious New Year's resolution was impossible to maintain. Depriving myself of all my favorite foods caused me to quit. "I'll just wait until next year," I would tell myself, knowing good and well I'd likely experience the same cycle in twelve months. After numerous resolutions of doing this, I started to question whether this insane cycle would ever end.

But on December 31, 2011, it was different. For the first time, I experienced what I never thought possible on a New Year's Eve: freedom.

Robynn and I had only lived out our concept for nine months, but let me tell ya, the feeling was incredible. I was able to enjoy bringing in 2012 without stuffing my face or feeling depressed that I would have to start a diet the very next day. In fact, I ate less on that night because I knew nothing would be off limits on January 1—or any day after.

Years have passed, and I continue to celebrate this late night holiday with the same refreshing feeling of freedom. No binging at midnight. No panic of having to start cold turkey on the first of January. In fact, as each December comes to an end, I can't help but reflect and give thanks for all the happiness I now have in my life. I no longer get wrapped up in crazy resolutions, but instead, I get excited about the new possibilities of the future. These days, I get to cherish every moment of ringing in a new year, because the next day is just business as usual.

Chapter 3 Take-Home Messages

Peace with Food:

✓ Helps track your progress by rating your actions and decisions.

✓ Builds your character.

✓ Gives you the simplicity your life has been longing for.

✓ Stops the feelings of deprivation. In return, it eliminates the spiraling-out-of-control behavior that causes you to binge.

✓ Empowers you to come up with what works best for your situation.

✓ Encourages finding what will keep you in the game. Discovering this will help increase your peace level, and as a result, your goals will be more attainable.

✓ Gives you the power to make a choice.

✓ Focuses on embracing the present moment.

✓ Thrives most when utilizing the support of others.

✓ Makes maintaining your weight easy. All you have to do is continue doing what you are already doing.

✓ Offers an amazing sense of freedom.

CHAPTER

4

Body

You Are Not Alone

Lara

When I met Robynn for the first time at the library, I remember
thinking how slim and fit she looked. I was at a healthy weight, but
as soon as I saw her, I recall thinking how I needed to start working
out and go on a diet. Little did I know she was exercising twice a
day and eating only vegetables for lunch. It wasn't until we became
closer friends that I was shocked to hear how often she felt
deprived and wasn't one hundred percent satisfied with her body.
From what I remembered, she looked awesome and had it all
together. Come to find out only half of that was true.

Have you ever found that no matter what your weight is, you
struggle with food and are unsatisfied with some area of your
body? Even when you have lost a significant amount of weight you

may feel overwhelmed with pressure to stay skinny, especially if people noticed and made a big deal about it.

The more people we talk to, women *and* men, the more we realize most humans struggle when it comes to body image or the number on the scale, regardless of their size. It is easy to believe that if you look thin and maintain your healthy BMI weight you are automatically happy and never struggle with food temptation. We think looking like that comes *easy*. Let us assure you, this is not true...well, at least not until you find peace with food, which will also give you peace with yourself.

Did you know that skinny people who lack peace think about food as much as overweight people? Even skinny people can be consumed with thoughts of food or a particular area of their body. You may tell yourself no one feels the same way you do, but that simply is not true. Most people deal with these same thoughts and frustrations throughout their lifetime, but rarely talk about it.

No person's life is as perfect as it appears, so give yourself a break. Stop comparing yourself to everyone else. Realize you both feel the same way, despite the fact that you look completely different. And above all, take comfort in knowing that no matter where you are in your journey, you are never alone.

Embrace Your Imperfect Self

There is no happier person than a truly content person.
~Joyce Meyer

Robynn

All right, I'll admit it. One area of my body I hated for years was my thighs. They are drumstick-shaped and not the pencil-shaped thighs you see in magazines. Because I carried around too much weight for much of my adult life, I actually thought I could have thighs that look like Carrie Underwood's. I love her thighs. I would rip out magazine pictures of models with similar shaped thighs and dream of the day I would have these beautifully sculpted works of art.

For years I had thought, "If I could just get down to my goal weight, I would have thin thighs." Then I began losing weight.

When I got down to my goal and my dream thighs didn't appear, I set my sights seven pounds lower. Still no thin thighs, so I set my sights even lower. At my lowest weight ever, my thighs still did not look like the ones in the magazines. You can imagine the disappointment I felt. *Ugh!*

At this point, I was at the bottom end of the normal BMI range. I could no longer handle the restrictions and totally rebelled against any diet that dared to tell me how to eat. The insane thing is I was actually quite happy with my body when I got a few pounds below my goal weight. But that wasn't enough. I wanted to have the perfect thighs. Talk about insanity! Thank goodness I eventually saw the light. My thighs are not as skinny as I had originally hoped, but I don't care anymore.

I'm amazed how I chased that rabbit trail for years. I wish I had said, "It is what it is" years ago. But the good news is now I know. I don't have to let it torment me any longer.

I know this story is crazy, but I share it because I have lived long enough to know countless others who hate either part or all of their body too. I'm all for changing what you can in a sensible way, but even as my situation illustrates, it's possible to go overboard. For many of us, the things we dislike about our bodies are things we have absolutely no control over—round face instead of oval, short legs, eyes too close together—you get the picture.

One piece of advice that Lara and I really like on this subject comes from author and speaker Sam Horn. In her book *What's Holding You Back?* she gives the approach "admire or aspire" as an alternative to comparing ourselves to others.[2]

When you see something in someone else that you like but either don't want to acquire (such as putting in the time and energy to be an Olympic swimmer) or you can't acquire (you love Celine Dion's voice, but can't carry a tune in a bucket), you appreciate and admire that quality by saying, "That's cool. I really admire them." Then you leave it at that. No remorse, no comparing. Just appreciating their gift to the world, knowing that you have something equally admirable.

On the other hand, you may see someone else's accomplishment or quality that you aspire to, such as earning your Master's degree or being patient with others. In this case you ask yourself, "How can I...?" and then take the necessary steps to reach that goal or acquire that quality. When tempted to compare yourself to others, instead admire or aspire.

What part of your body do you wish looked different? This is not exclusive to women. The first time I read this vignette to my husband, Scott, he told me that he, too, had been dissatisfied with his thighs back in the day. Except that he wished his were bigger. Being a weightlifter and even winning a gold medal in the Junior Olympics, he said the majority of other weightlifters had bulky thighs. His weren't as big as he had wanted. Go figure!

The moral of this story is: Enjoy your imperfect self. Doing so will help you enjoy your life and those people and blessings you already have.

Accept What You Can't Change

God grant me the serenity to accept the things I cannot change, the courage to change the things I can, and the wisdom to know the difference.
~Reinhold Niebuhr

There comes a time when you need to look at your life, your whole life, and see an accurate picture of who you are. This includes your:

- Strengths
- Weaknesses
- Body (height, musculature, metabolism)
- Relationships (or lack of)
- Passions (those things that stir your soul)
- Resources of time, money, and opportunities

This is also where you face the 800-pound gorilla in the room and confront him once and for all.

The 800-pound gorilla is the area of your body you don't like and can't change. For Lara, it was not having a smaller upper body. For Robynn, it was her drumstick thighs. Remember, she wanted the Carrie Underwood version? Even at the lower end of their weight ranges, these areas of their body were larger than what they preferred. Some things you won't be able to change, but there is something you can do about the way you feel.

If you want to move forward, there comes a time when you must look that gorilla square in the eyes and say, "Good riddance." Slam the door behind you, and leave that nemesis for good. When you do, you won't believe the freedom that comes because you dared to confront that crazy ape.

Face Reality in the Mirror

Face reality as it is, not as it was or as you wish it to be.
~Jack Welch

Lara

And there I stood, staring at my figure in the reflection of my mirror. As my eyes made their way up to my face, all I could see was a look of confusion. The compliments I received earlier that day kept running through my mind: "You look amazing! What have you done to look so fit?"

Who were they talking about? Was I one hundred percent sure they were talking to me? Surely it was a dream. It had to be, because when I see me, I don't see what they were talking about.

The disconnect happens when we can't see what actually is. We are told we look thinner, but our eyes see a flabby body in need of losing a few more pounds. If someone says we are pretty, all we see are the wrinkles around our eyes and sun damage on our cheeks. We don't merely tell ourselves these negative things, we truly see them that way. This is exactly why you see super skinny women in the magazines who say they are fat. They are suffering from the disconnect.

Have you ever gone through old photos? You may have found yourself saying, "Wow. I looked good. I can't believe I thought I was overweight back then." We have done this too, and the lesson has been learned. There is a disconnect between reality and what you see in the mirror. For that reason, we suggest taking a picture. It is our easiest solution to the disconnect. A photo not only documents where you are (in true photographic form) but helps you see what actually is.

Just to be sure, I put this to the test. One afternoon, there I stood again, looking in the mirror with disgust. Enough was enough, so I grabbed the camera, put it on auto-take and posed. (The door was closed, of course. I would have been mortified if someone walked in and wondered what in the world I was doing.)

Sure enough, my jaw dropped when I flipped through the pictures I'd just taken. I was amazed at how much thinner I looked compared to how I'd felt looking in the mirror a few minutes before.

The mirror, scale, or even clothing are some of the things that can work against you as much as for you. They are all capable of letting you slide into yet another insane cycle. Stop the madness, my friend. Don't base your mood on one outfit or one glance in the mirror. Find other ways to see yourself in a different light. When you do, the results are often better than you think.

Robynn

The opposite of this can be true as well. I remember one time I saw a television commercial in which a lady was sharing her weight loss success story. Her motivation for going on a diet was seeing a picture of herself at her friend's wedding. On the television screen flashed a picture of this lady when she was grossly overweight.

I was amazed that it took that picture for her to realize her need to lose weight. What was going on in her mind the day of the wedding as she dressed in front of the mirror? Apparently, it was not that she needed to go on a diet. That revelation would come as she saw herself in pictures days later.

As obvious as this was to me, being the outsider, I felt compassion for this lady. I, too, have experienced the disconnect with the mirror and have been jolted into reality by seeing myself in a picture.

For some reason, a picture can make a statement the mirror simply can't. So, again, get out the camera and take the picture. It lasts longer and does a better job at revealing what really is.

Obsessing for No Good Reason

Lara

In college, I took voice lessons every semester as part of my music education degree. In order to graduate, I was required to present a senior recital. This concert consisted of a solo performance lasting over thirty minutes. Just the idea of singing that long makes a person's throat hurt, and standing alone in front of a crowd with all eyes on you can cause even more panic!

My voice professor told me, "When you are up on stage, don't worry about the audience and what they are thinking. Believe it or not, they won't be thinking about *you*. People are too consumed thinking about themselves. They won't focus solely on you for very long."

I had never given it much thought, but what he said seemed to be true. When you step inside someone's new house, you typically think to yourself how you wish you had the same house or perhaps you compare it to your own home. If you see a child acting out in the grocery store, your thoughts immediately focus on how you, "hope *my* kids don't do that to me when I'm in public." Rarely do we pick apart the other person without eventually turning the focus back on ourselves.

The same applies to body image. Despite the stress of singing in front of a crowd, the one thing I was paranoid about during my recital was how chunky my arms looked in my performance gown. If I had asked every person in the audience what they were thinking as I stood on stage, I could almost guarantee no one would have mentioned my chunky arms.

We become so paranoid with certain areas of our body we forget that no one thinks about our bodies the way we do. If you lose weight, people look at you and think, "Oh, I need to hit the gym." The focus on you may only be for a second, but they are mostly thinking about how *they* need to eat better or improve a certain part of their physique.

So next time you are in a panic over a couple of pounds increase, or however much it may be, remind yourself that no one else is fretting over it like you are.

Keep calm and carry on. There is no need to obsess over something no one else is even thinking about.

Look and Feel Your Best

Once you begin to experience peace with food in your life, you will begin to see that it has a ripple effect in other areas too.

One of the areas in which our concept made a big impact on us was in our appearance. Until discovering this concept, we were hit-and-miss at looking our best. If we were out in public, we most likely presented ourselves well. However, at home, chances are you would find us wearing sweats, no makeup, and hair undone.

But as we began to walk in peace, we began to look at ourselves differently and adopted the policy of always looking our best. That doesn't mean we don't wear sweats or comfy clothes or even pull our hair up in a ponytail, but we always strive to look presentable, wearing what we consider to be cute, comfy clothes with our hair done and some makeup applied.

A good rule of thumb is this: If someone came to your door unannounced, would you feel confident or embarrassed by the way you looked?

Another part of this equation is finding out what type of clothes and hair styles look best on you. And again, this happens with trial and error. If you are into fashion, makeup, and hair, this will come easy. If this is not your forte, enlist a friend who is good with such things.

Along with getting their advice and input, have your friend take pictures of you in different clothing and hairstyles. Make sure you get pictures of your backside as well. This may sound funny, but many times you may think you look great only to discover your backside is not as forgiving as what you saw looking in the mirror.

Start today by banishing what doesn't look good on you and/or make you feel happy. Usually a size up makes you look slimmer. And when selecting your style in hair, makeup, wardrobe, and other areas of your appearance, always keep this in mind:

Maximize your assets and minimize your liabilities.

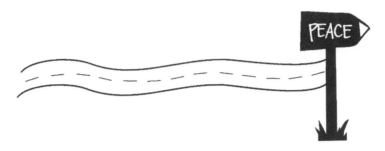

C. The Boutique

Appearance—What makes you look and feel the best?

- _____
- _____
- _____
- _____
- _____
- _____
- _____

Hair:

	Where I Get Compliments	What I Like Best on Me
Color		
Cut		
Style		
Length		

Wardrobe:

	Where I Get Compliments	What I Like Best on Me
Jeans		
Dress Pants		
Skirts		
Dresses		
Tops		
Comfy Clothes		
Casual Clothes		
Dress Clothes		

Lara: Snug work-out clothes, flattering clothes like my skinny jeans with a pair of boots, and a fitted T-shirt. Definitely, no oversized T-shirts! As far as hair is concerned, I feel the best when I get my hair highlighted and professionally styled. If I start the day putting my hair up in a cute ponytail and applying some makeup, my likelihood of eating better, staying active, and feeling good increases dramatically. As I said, I am a big believer in always wearing clothes that make you feel and look great, no matter what size you are. Some clothes may make you feel good but don't necessarily flatter. As long as they make you feel better about yourself, wear them. At the very least, you could wear them around the house where you are most comfortable. I wear workout pants that are tight-fitting, and although I am far from looking like a workout guru, it motivates me to eat better and be more active.

Robynn: I actually love fashion, so that's a hard one, but I especially love blue jeans, heels, cute workout clothes, and getting dressed up. One summer I weighed at the upper range of my BMI. I felt cruddy about myself. Lara talked me into buying jean shorts that were flattering at that weight. No, I didn't love the way I looked in them; however, they were more flattering than anything else I had in my closet. I am so glad Lara talked me into buying those shorts because I got so much use out of them. Although I wasn't at my goal weight, they made me feel the best at the size I was then.

Chapter 4 Take-Home Messages

✓No person's life is as perfect as it appears.

✓Use the approach "admire or aspire" as an alternative to comparing ourselves to others.

✓To live at peace you must accept once and for all what you cannot change.

✓The mirror is not always the best indicator of how you really look. Next time, consider taking a picture.

✓Don't waste time fretting over something no one else is thinking about.

✓Find out what makes you look and feel the best.

CHAPTER

5

Mind

Know Yourself

Know yourself to improve yourself.
~Auguste Comte

If you want peace with food, you must quit trying to fit into everyone else's "box" and, as the cliché goes, just be yourself. It sounds simple, but unfortunately it isn't. If it were, we'd all be doing it! But if you take a look around, you will see countless people (maybe yourself included) who are attempting to live their lives the way someone else is living theirs. They assume if a particular diet plan, parenting technique, or financial approach works for someone else, it must work for everyone. They eagerly enlist, give it their best shot, and become disappointed when their actions don't produce the results they hoped for.

French philosopher Auguste Comte said, "Know yourself to improve yourself." Socrates put it this way: "The unexamined life is not worth living."

Great advice. But something we don't always do, especially in our hectic lives. Besides, it can be a bit messy and inconvenient. After all, maybe we will find something we don't like. Maybe we will be faced with a character trait that we would rather not acknowledge. Or maybe we just don't have the time to really delve into the deepest parts of us: our hopes, ours fears, our dreams.

Maybe we don't want to take the time to know ourselves because then we will be forced to speak up and perhaps rock the boat. Maybe we will have to confront or challenge the status quo. That may be the down-side, but there is also an up-side to digging deeper: Knowing yourself gives you direction and clarity. It acts as a compass, pointing you in the direction you should go. Knowing yourself also makes life easier in that it eliminates options and makes your choices clearer...and trust us, that is a good thing.

In living with peace, whether that be with food, finances, relationships, or whatever it may be, you need to know yourself. What are your preferences? Your likes? Dislikes? What gives you peace? What leaves you with that pit in your stomach? What do you value most?

How well do you know yourself?

In this book we will discuss the many different aspects of your life such as weight, exercise, food, habits, and temptation. To have direction in each of these areas, self-knowledge is not only helpful, but necessary.

Here's a list of questions to help you know yourself in these areas. They may not all be appropriate for each scenario, but consider using these questions any time you want to learn more about yourself in an area you want to improve.

- What is your greatest heart's desire regarding_____?
- What makes your heart sing regarding_____?
- What is your greatest fear regarding_____?
- What discourages you or defeats you regarding _____?
- What one thing would you change about_____?
- What do you value most in the area of_____?

- What are your gifts and talents regarding
  _____?
- What comes easy for you, but not necessarily for others
  in the area of _____?
- What is difficult for you, but not necessarily for others
  in the area of _____?
- What motivates you regarding_____?
- What do you like in regards to _____?
- What do you dislike in regards to _____?
- What would you do if you knew you were guaranteed
  success in regards to _____?
- What would life look like if it were perfect in regards to
  _____?

These questions got us started, but we didn't stop there. We're still asking ourselves questions and searching for ways we can be better and do better.

When you really know yourself—your roles, preferences, strengths, weaknesses, tendencies, and all those things that make you uniquely you—then you can ease up on yourself and do the things that work best for you. No more trying to squeeze into someone else's box. No more trying to fit a square peg into a round hole. No more trying to please others.

If you've been attempting to fit into someone else's mold, you may have found that it only leaves you feeling uncomfortable with who you are. If so, free yourself by living your life in a way that is designed for you. Once you have the freedom to accept yourself and all your idiosyncrasies, you are ready to embrace your life. Then, and only then, you will be able to enjoy the one and only you.

Determine Your Value

Robynn

An apple-green vase. There it sits, surrounded by white dishes in a completely white kitchen. I love how it draws your eye as if to say, "Look at me." Although it was created as a vase, I don't like to use it as one. Instead, I want it to stay right where it is. That vase is special to me. It is valuable. It's my souvenir from a trip to Europe, where Scott and I traveled a year after our wedding. It came from a glass factory in Venice, and when I saw it in the store window, I knew this was the one. To me it is irreplaceable—a one-of-a-kind piece of art that is valuable. Very, very valuable.

This vase makes me think of people, specifically the ones struggling to find happiness in their lives. I guess I know, because I've been there. I know how value gets distorted when you don't feel good about yourself.

Let's say Lara and I gave you two $10 bills. The first one was ripped, written on, crinkled, and worn. The second was brand new, crisp, clean, and unused. If we asked which one has greater value, what would you answer? Would you say the second because it is clean and crisp? Would the first bill have less value when you went to the grocery store because it was tattered? The obvious answer is "No." Although they appear very different on the outside, they are equally worth $10.

How you see yourself will determine the life you live, the path you take, and how you view yourself and your world. So, what is your value? Your answer to this question will be telling. Do you consider yourself valuable?

The issue of value is critical because your perception of your worth is the eyepiece you will be looking through. If the eyepiece is distorted, everything you look at will be distorted.

Now let's talk about value. Value has to do with worth. We could actually interchange the two words and ask you, what's your worth?

Value = Worth

On a scale of one to ten, your worth, your value, is a 10. Regardless of your condition, regardless your past, regardless your life, you are a 10. Period.

Maybe you think you are worthless. Not so. Maybe you think because you failed miserably or because others failed you miserably, you don't deserve to be anything but a second-class citizen. However, if you are to live the life created for you, it is vitally important that you see yourself as the incredibly valuable and unique person you are.

Once you discover you are valuable—a perfect 10—you have a choice to make. Will you fulfill your potential and live with purpose?

Choose a Purposeful or Purposeless Life

If you have felt hopeless, hold on! Wonderful changes are going to happen in your life as you begin to live it on purpose.
~Rick Warren

Understanding your value is crucial because people who don't feel valuable don't fulfill their purpose. They don't believe they have a purpose. However, when you settle the value issue for good, you are ready to pursue your purpose. You make the choice:

1. Be the valuable person you are and be purposeful.
2. Be the valuable person you are and be purposeless.

Using the same analogy we used in the previous vignette, imagine we gave two people a $10 bill. One person took their bill and buried it while the other put it to use by making a transaction.

If we were to trace the 18-month life cycle of the $10 bill, it may circle the globe. Just think about the interesting things and people it would see along the way.

If the $10 bill goes through thirty or so transactions in its life cycle, it is still worth $10, yet it has multiplied itself significantly. Changing hands thirty times means the bill has conducted $300 worth of transactions!

Compare that $10 to the one still buried in the ground. Although the value of each $10 bill remains the same, the one buried did not fulfill its purpose. However, the one interchanged many times lived up to its potential.

These $10 bills represent our lives. Our value is a 10. There is nothing we or anyone can do to change that. We decide the quality of our life by choosing to be either purposeful or purposeless.

Do What Successful People Do

Successful people think about what they want and how to get that. Unsuccessful people think about what they don't want and who is to blame for their problems and difficulties.
~Brian Tracy

Maybe you have struggled much of your life doubting yourself. How do you change your opinion to one of belief? How do you change the negative habit of doubt to one of positive expectation?

Do what successful people do.

In studying the lives of successful people, we have seen the power of positive affirmations. *Affirmation* probably isn't a word that most people hear every day. An affirmation is basically a positive statement about yourself that you say out loud on a regular basis.

This is important because of the impact this activity has on your mind. It is like a self-fulfilled prophesy coming to pass. As you visualize the person you desire to be, and then verbalize these desires, your mind begins to go to work—your actions begin to adjust to this new picture your mind has been given.

Sound difficult? It's not. Writing your own personal affirmations is actually quite easy. The following list will get you started:

- Visualize the person that you desire to be. To create your own affirmations, you need to know what you want to do, be, and have. What's important to you? What do you dream about? Where would you like to be in a year? Five years? Ten years? What does your future body look like in the mirror? How much do you weigh? How do you feel?
- Grab a notebook, 3x5 index cards, or your computer to record your affirmations.
- Begin each affirmation with the words "I am…"
- Put your affirmations in a positive light, rather than a negative one. (Choose "I am eating healthy…" rather than "I am not eating unhealthy…")

- Place the verb in each affirmation in the present progressive tense by using -ing. ("I am living at peace with food..." rather than "I live at peace with food...") This signifies to your brain that you are presently doing the positive action.
- Keep it simple.

Here are some examples:

- "I am living a self-controlled and disciplined life."
- "I am making wise choices in my eating and exercising."
- "I am improving daily at not wasting my calories."
- "I am happily maintaining a healthy weight."
- "I am living my dream of having a healthy body, healthy relationships, and peace of mind."

Once you compile your affirmations, begin saying them daily, multiple times if possible. The more you hear yourself say them, the sooner you begin believing them. As you say your affirmations, see yourself as the person in each statement. If your affirmation speaks of being confident, see yourself acting in a confident manner as you relate to others. If it speaks of being self-controlled, see yourself having self-control in the situations where you typically lack this quality. If it speaks of being patient, see yourself being patient as you deal with the people and circumstances that tend to rattle you.

As you practice the skill of daily speaking your affirmations, you'll start seeing yourself as the person you are professing to be.

Another method you may find helpful is creating a vision board. A vision board is a place where you compile pictures and words that describe what you want your future to look like. You can create your vision board on a physical bulletin board, in a notebook, or on a space on your wall. Another option is to use an online resource like a private blog or Pinterest (www.pinterest.com). The vision board's purpose is to inspire you to see yourself as the person you want to be. As we said, this is very powerful, because seeing a picture of things you desire has a positive effect on your brain.

As you begin collecting pictures and images, include words describing how you wish to be: confident, courageous, self-controlled, stable, persistent. Include pictures of clothes you want to wear at your desired weight, the places you would like to go, and visuals depicting the emotions of peace and joy you will experience as you progress in your journey. See yourself as that person and little by little your growth will begin to appear.

Go ahead and start dreaming! Visualize your life the way you want it to be, and before you know it, you'll begin to see it transpire.

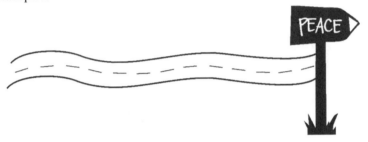

D. Lookout Point

Affirmations—List your affirmations regarding peace with food and a healthy body.

- _____
- _____
- _____
- _____
- _____
- _____
- _____

Lara: "I am living a self-controlled and disciplined life. I am making wise choices in my eating and exercising."

Robynn: "I am improving daily at not wasting my calories. I am happily maintaining a healthy weight."

Get Real with Yourself

If it doesn't challenge you, it doesn't change you.
~Fred DeVito

They say misery loves company. For some that may be true, but in our experience with being out-of-control in our eating, misery was, well…a great motivator.

Misery motivated us to take a good look at our lives and be willing to do whatever it required to make a change. It inspired us to refuse to sit on the sidelines and instead to be more present in the game of life.

Throughout this process we had to sit down and have many "hard reality" talks. We have included some of those talks below.

Talk #1—Moment of Truth: Want to weigh ten pounds less than what is reasonable and healthy for your height and body type? Maybe you are putting off peace with food because now is not a convenient time, even though your sanity depends on it and your quality of life stinks.

Sounds like it's time for a reality check. Look yourself in the mirror, ditch the excuses, and honestly assess where you are and where you are headed if you don't make the changes now.

Talk #2—The Mole Hill: Boy, we humans can be melodramatic. You have a bad weekend or gain a few pounds and think it's the end of the world. Instead of making a mountain out of a mole hill, why not take a better approach and have a heart-to-heart with yourself. Are things really as bad as you are making them out to be? Instead of looking at the glass as half-empty, consider taking the opposite approach by learning from the experience.

We wrote this book by recording all our successes—but even more importantly, our failures. Over time we could see how beneficial it was to look at our failures as positives. With each step backward, we actually took five steps forward by learning how to handle the situation better next time. Thomas J. Watson, founder of IBM, says,

If you want to increase your success rate,
double your failure rate.

With that kind of attitude, you don't have to be afraid of failure. Instead, you can use your failures to your advantage. Let them motivate you to make the changes necessary for success. To get started, have a "hard reality" talk with yourself and take one step closer to your goal.

Prioritize Your Life

Step with care and great tact. And remember that Life's a Great Balancing Act.
~Dr. Seuss

So you have a "hard reality" talk with yourself about your physical condition and then promise to make a change. You may say something like, "Ok, I'm going to be the best me I can physically be." You then enlist in a strict plan consisting of eating only so-called healthy foods and commit to working out for hours. Your focus is only on your physical appearance at the expense of other aspects of your life.

Remember, you are a complex being and you must look at the whole picture. When you set physical goals, see them in the context of all those other areas of life: your marriage, children, relationships, responsibilities, and your faith.

Imagine contestants in a cooking show with limited budgets to prepare a meal. They fill their shopping carts with ingredients, only to see they have overspent. This requires them to go through the cart and take out ingredients that are least important. Sure, they would like to keep the whole cart of groceries, but because that's not possible, and they have the final dish in mind, they choose to keep only the most important items.

One piece of advice is to invest the least amount of time for the maximum results. In other words, get the biggest bang for your buck! And while this concept does not apply to everything, it should at least help you to prioritize.

If eating moderately and exercising five times a week will help you lose seven pounds a month, we wouldn't consider it a wise choice to exercise twice as much to lose an extra two pounds in the same amount of time. You have to prioritize and determine what people and activities are going to get the greater part of your attention.

Certainly your health and well-being are important, but don't place all your focus on a single aspect of your life at the expense of your relationships. When you are on your deathbed, you will not be spending your final hour thinking about how you should have spent more time at the gym so your arms could be more defined or chiseled. You will, however, be focused on the people in your life and whether you made an impact on others. So see the big picture.

By using peace with food to reach your weight loss goal, you don't have to sacrifice your life in order to get there. Whether or not you want to admit it, your time on earth is limited. Use it wisely because once it's gone, it's gone.

Reset

Robynn

Does this scenario sound familiar to you: you eat more than you had planned and feel so discouraged you throw in the towel? Did what started as a few hundred extra calories then become a few thousand or more? We hope by now you are getting the picture— eating in a way that gives peace is a lifelong process resulting in greater degrees of success with every step you take. And as with everything in life, things aren't always going to be perfect.

Let's say you went out with a friend for dinner and a movie. You ended up spending more than you planned at dinner and the movie you saw turned out to be a total waste of time and money. Would you cut your losses, or would you go out and spend an extra $1,000 because you blew $50?

Now unless you have a major spending issue (which is probably the topic for another book), your answer was likely to cut your losses and move on.

If this is the most reasonable and likely response, why don't we use this approach when it comes to food? Think about it for a moment. You overeat by a little, or even a lot, but instead of cutting your losses you consume an extra, 2,000-4,000 calories or more. This is obviously insanity, but it is a habit, and old habits die hard.

To stop the insanity, make a new habit—the habit of hitting the reset button. And here's how you do it:

Make a choice.

What one or two habits, if you possessed them, would revolutionize your life where peace with food is concerned? That is the question I asked myself, and it's a question that took me a year and a half to answer. But when I finally did, I came to the following conclusion: Have the skill to get back on track after a slip-up instead of giving up for the rest of the day.

This was crucial to my success because many times a little slip-up would result in my spiraling out of control for days, weeks, or even months. It was unbelievable. I was baffled at how a little mistake, such as eating an extra 400 calorie dessert, caused so much turmoil. I knew there had to be a better way and that better way was to make a choice and reset.

We don't always do this perfectly, but here's what resetting looks like for us: We cut our losses and try to spend the rest of the day eating like we normally would. We don't make up for a slip-up by skipping a meal unless we are full and won't feel deprived by doing so.

Before discovering peace with food, I was still in the dieting/depriving mindset. I was determined that the easiest way to nip a slip-up in the bud was to go without food for a few days. Yes, I would actually not eat for a couple of days so I could get back down to the weight I was at before the slip-up.

Going without food robbed me of my happiness and always left me hungry. I became determined to learn how to get back on track after a slip-up, even if it took the rest of my life.

When I finally said good-bye to dieting, I decided no matter how many times I messed up, I would no longer deprive myself of food to lose weight. Instead I would learn how to get a clean slate immediately. I was aware there might be a possible gain the next day because I went over my ideal allotment of food for the day, but I was prepared to remind myself that it is target practice and I am in this for the long haul.

Hitting reset may be the single most important skill to have in your repertoire for rebounding from mistakes. It is for me anyway. And it will take time, patience, and self-control.

Are you ready to give yourself a second chance at this very moment? Once you develop this skill you won't need a new day, month, or year to get a fresh start. Instead, you have an incredible ability to hit reset at any given moment.

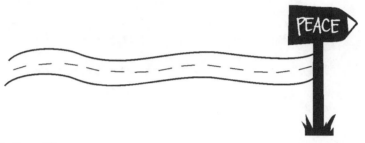

E. Stop Sign
Resetting—How can you use resetting to your advantage when it comes to food, exercise, or your weight on the scale?

- _____
- _____
- _____
- _____
- _____
- _____
- _____

Lara: Not only do I use the reset button with food, but I use it with exercise. In the past if I had a goal to exercise Monday through Friday and wasn't able to work out on Tuesday, I would stress out. I felt like I had to squeeze that missed workout in my already busy schedule. Sometimes I would give up altogether and wait until Monday to start over. Nowadays, if I had the same goal but needed to miss a day, I would reset each morning so I don't feel like I am always playing catch-up. I am a big believer in starting fresh.

Lara and Robynn: Have a "hard reality" talk with ourselves, call or text each other, get busy doing something else, reassess our goals, and get right back on track.

Pitch the All-or-Nothing Mindset

Don't use all-or-nothing thinking. Take each day as its own day, and don't worry about it if you mess up one day. The most important thing you can do is just get back up on the horse.
~Henry Cloud

Lara

Some days I wonder what happened to me. The girl who grew up believing when she was a Mom there would never be a pile of mail at the end of the dinner table...The girl who would always be able to see the bottom of the laundry basket because "it's not that hard to quickly throw in a load of dirty laundry to stay caught up." Yeah. Right.

I had a typical Type A personality—a far cry from a procrastinator, driven by a to-do list, punctual, organized, passionate. Yes, I was all of those things, and to some degree I still am. But more than anything, I was this: all-or-nothing.

I had an idea in my mind of how things should go, and if it didn't happen a certain way, then I might as well forget it. If I couldn't stay caught up on my mail and laundry, then I might as well clear my schedule, ignore the kids for a day, and put all my focus on marking tasks off my to-do list.

After about five years of living this way, I learned this mindset was a never-ending battle. I was always beating myself up and missing out on precious moments of life because I was so fixated on the way things should go. I thought if I did everything by the book, then things should fall perfectly into place. Boy was I wrong.

Fast forward a bit, and I'm still the same girl, but I think I have found the new me. I still have Type A tendencies, but God has sanded my rough edges and taught me to relax a little. I pitched the all-or-nothing mindset. I'm now the girl (and Mom) who realizes at 4:00 in the afternoon I haven't brushed my teeth yet. Instead of feeling guilty about admitting my failures at the upcoming dentist appointment, I am happy that at least I remembered. *Wink*. I'm the girl who catches myself turning to food in a stressful moment and six-hundred calories later stops to realize that food won't make my stress go away. At this moment I hit reset and don't beat myself up over what just happened. I'm the girl who will take what I can get even if it isn't perfect. I'm able to let go on those early mornings I get up to work, only to hear a little kid pitter-patter down the hall and start my day two hours earlier than expected. I adjust. I savor. I now live for those moments because I understand that peace happens when I stop trying to control everything.

Letting go of the all-or-nothing mindset will take your life to a whole new level. It has for me anyway. Although I wonder what happened to the old me, I am actually grateful I never found her…because the new me has more joy in her life than I ever thought possible.

Robynn

From the time I was a kid, I struggled with perfectionism. I remember at a young age practicing the piano. My system for practicing was to start at the beginning, and as soon as I made a mistake, I had to start the song all over again.

The insanity of this method is clear. What I needed to work on were the areas where I had made mistakes, not the first few measures of the song.

As I got older, I continued to be plagued by my all-or-nothing mindset: throwing up my hands and not studying in college because I realized it was impossible to read all the pages assigned by the professor. I even quit college basketball after my sophomore year because I couldn't practice the five-hour-a-day requirement I put on myself.

It saddens me to think of all the opportunities I wasted because of this faulty belief system. And even though I knew my thinking was flawed, I couldn't seem to break free from it.

What really helped me overcome this mindset was recognizing two approaches to take in life. They are what I call the lottery approach and the target approach. Here's a breakdown:

The Lottery Approach
- You either win it or you don't.
- The chances of you winning are extremely slim.
- There's not much you can do to increase your chances of winning.
- If you fail (which you usually do) there is no way to increase your chances of winning next time.

The Target Approach
- You can win every time because winning isn't about hitting the center of the target, it's about gaining the skills that will help you be more precise. Someone could be lucky and hit the center target on the first attempt, but this doesn't mean they have the skill to do it again.
- You are in complete control of increasing your success by exercising determination, hard work, and skill.
- Failure isn't a negative in this game if you take on the role of a student learning to improve your game.

The lottery approach is an all-or-nothing approach and its focus is the destination. As a result, you never get to fully enjoy life because you spend so little time fully engaged in life. The target approach, on the other hand, strives for continual improvement and growth. Because its focus is the journey, you get to enjoy your life daily.

Give Yourself Grace

How's that working for you?
~Dr. Phil McGraw

The torture chamber. We spend so much time there because that's where diets end up taking us. It's part of the insane cycle—the habit of repeatedly torturing ourselves with some of the following:

• Depriving ourselves of the food we want the most.
• Subjecting ourselves to unnecessary temptation.
• Being confined by strict rules.
• Having an all-or-nothing perfectionist mindset that causes us to give up when we make the slightest mistake.
• Hoping (and expecting) to look like an airbrushed model in a magazine.

Humor us just a bit and at least consider there might be a better way to reach your weight goal than living in the torture chamber. After all, there's no peace there.

Diets overlook an important quality: *grace*. That's because diet dictators try to make us believe that if we're committed enough, disciplined enough, and focused enough, we will lose weight on their plan.

We just have to wonder about the people writing those books. Do they really live by the rules they are prescribing? Have they ever walked a mile in our shoes? Has weight ever been an issue for them?

Even if they do eat according to the rules they set forth, why are they so convinced their rules work for everyone else? The answer is probably quite simple: because their plan comes so easy to them, they believe everyone else has the peace to follow it to a T.

Instead, we ask that you give yourself grace. In other words, be kind to yourself. This isn't giving yourself permission to cast off all restraint and go off the deep end. It's loving yourself enough to put an end to all those crazy things we do to lose the unwanted pounds. It's refusing to believe the insidious lies of our culture attempting to define us by how we look, resisting the pressure to conform to their ideals.

We are all different. What works for one doesn't always work for another, and although many of these people are well meaning and want to help others, their methods are flawed. They don't give grace—the very thing that helps us get to where we need to go.

Understanding the necessity of giving grace to yourself, as well as others, is so important because this journey is a learning process, and it takes time. Beating yourself up over your mistakes won't give peace and will slow your progress.

Throughout the process, whether you are consistently hitting the target or not, you'll need grace. So stop the torture. Enough already! It's time to enjoy some grace.

Assess the Influence of Your Relationships

The people you surround yourself with influence your behaviors, so choose friends who have healthy habits.
~Dan Buettner

Lara

If you want your life to head in a certain direction, you'll get the best results by surrounding yourself with people who live the life you are striving for.

My husband and I have found that making improvements—whether in our marriage, finances, parenting, or how we treat other people—is much easier when we hang out with others who push us to improve in these areas. We don't necessarily have conversations about these specific subjects, however simply hanging around them and observing their actions keeps us in check.

This can be true in the area of eating as well. Your relationships are a huge factor to consider because, like it or not, people can influence the way you eat.

Almost any time family gathers, food is involved. This can be fun and enjoyable, but also difficult if those around you have a different mindset concerning food.

If your family is not controlled in their eating, you likely won't be able to eat like them and have peace with food. Some families have an unhealthy relationship with food. It is the center of their lives and they eat excessively, indulgently, and in an unhealthy manner.

With that said, high calorie meals are not always a negative in families. If you have a teenage athlete or a spouse whose work involves manual labor, they may be burning enough calories to allow them to consume much more food without gaining weight than your own activity level allows.

Whether the influences are good or bad, it is natural to model their behavior when you are around them. Tough choices have to be made regarding eating events or the type of activities you do when you get together. This can be extremely difficult, but in order to have peace in this area, you may need to be creative or volunteer a non-food activity if you are around these people often.

For example, many times friends want to plan a night out. If they ask you for ideas, use those opportunities to suggest activities that won't put you in a situation of temptation. You could pick a time of day, before or after mealtimes, so eating won't be on the agenda. Or if a parent asks you to set up a play date, suggest meeting at the track to walk or do something that doesn't revolve around food. More often than not, they will follow your lead if you initiate it first.

How can you create eating situations that allow you to be with loved ones without sacrificing peace with food? It can be done, but may require you to think outside the box.

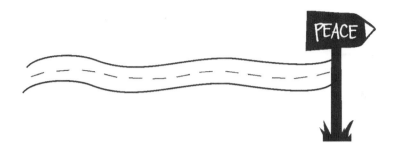

F. Picnic Table

Influence of Others—What is the culture of your relationships regarding food or self-image? Include events that negatively impact your feelings regarding food, eating, or your body.

- _____
- _____
- _____
- _____
- _____
- _____

Lara: It is on very rare occasions that I feel like my friends or family insists on me eating something I don't want. Years ago, my husband and I would talk one another into finishing off a meal (even if we were full) any time there was food left in the serving dish. Now that we both live at peace with food that conversation never comes up! We both know we aren't going to waste calories after experiencing closure by finishing our plate of food. We are also more likely to hold one another accountable to stop eating when we are full. And because we enjoy leftovers, I usually talk myself into saving the food back so I can enjoy it again the next day.

Lara and Robynn: Ironically both of our husbands love cooking and trying new recipes. Because their food is so delicious it would be easy to overeat, but fortunately our husbands also know when to stop, which makes it easier for us.

Choose Peace over Panic

Do not pray for easy lives. Pray to be stronger men.
~John F. Kennedy

Boy, do we wish there was a fix-all solution when it comes to being at peace with food. You probably remember the Staples® commercial showcasing the big red "Easy Button" that fixes any problem. It would be nice to have one of these gadgets in everyday life so something difficult could instantly become *easy*.

Unfortunately, it's not that simple. Life is challenging. And contrary to popular belief, life does not have to be easy for us to have fulfilled, contented, and abundant lives. We can endure trials and tough times and do it with grit, determination, and joy.

Each one of us has a choice to make. We have to decide whether we will choose the peace button or the panic button when things don't go as planned.

We are very familiar with the panic button because we have pushed it more times than we can count. *Sigh.* Maybe you've experienced this as well. You know all about those feelings—they scream at you like an out-of-control child, sending you over the edge and causing you to frantically hang on by your fingernails.

It is during times like this that you must sit yourself down and have a reality check. Maybe you are panicking because you gained an extra five pounds over the holidays. When you are learning to live at peace with food you will take small steps day in and day out to become successful rather than panic and do something extreme that you'll later regret.

The panic button is always available. Fortunately, so is the peace button. Do yourself a favor, choose the second.

Recognize an "Off" Day

Lara

If you lived in my house, you would know it is a regular occurrence that I frantically search for my skinny jeans. Some days, no matter what I try on, I just feel uncomfortable. Even the jeans that made me feel skinny the day before can become my pair of fat jeans the very next day.

The real reason I become frustrated has little to do with how I feel in my clothes and more to do with how I feel in general. I've come to realize that even if I'm eating right and having peace with food and exercise, there will still be days I won't feel like a million bucks when I slip (okay squeeze) into my blue jeans. That's just the way it goes sometimes. No matter what we do or how great we are tackling our goals, our body is going to feel different from what we think it should. Do you ever have days like that? (Don't leave me hanging... I would be devastated if you said I wasn't normal!)

So what do I do in the meantime? I allow myself a free pass. I don't panic. I don't do anything extreme with my eating. I just keep doing what I'm doing and don't let my emotions get the best of me.

When we temporarily feel extra fat or lethargic, it is easy to cave to a quick-fix diet. Either that or we go to the completely opposite end of the spectrum and allow ourselves to binge in hopes of masking how we feel. It is easy to get sucked into the insane cycle at this point because, either way, your jump is going to be a disaster...unless you don't jump at all. So next time you find yourself feeling uneasy with your emotions, ride out the wave. Like all things, this feeling too shall pass. Before you know it, your skinny jeans will turn up, and you'll be thankful you didn't do anything to disrupt your path to peace.

Take Advantage of a Rainy Day

The best way out of a difficulty is through it.
~Will Rogers

Lara

Rainy days are sometimes associated with being unproductive and depressing. Sunny days, on the other hand, are usually connected with being motivated and feeling good.

Experiencing the funk is very comparable to a rainy day. Sometimes the forecast shows thunderstorms for an entire week and other times it only lasts a day or a few hours. This is why having a pep talk with yourself will be so crucial during your funk days. You may feel like it will last forever, but remind yourself—realistically—it doesn't last long.

Even though most people think of rainy days as being bad, I've learned how to make them work to my favor. I was determined to turn a negative day into one with positive outcomes. Rainy days force me to be inside, so I utilize this time by snuggling up with my kids, catching up on scrapbooking, or doing some deep cleaning around the house. Those things can be rewarding, but I won't want to be doing those types of activities once the weather turns nice. I am always excited when the sun decides to pop out, but I don't feel guilty for lost time because I know the rainy days were not wasted.

If you allow yourself to eat as much as you want or to stop exercising whenever you're in a funk, you'll be further behind when your emotions get back on track. But if you push through a funk by riding out the rainy day, you'll be way ahead of the game once the sun begins to shine.

Keep Calm and Carry On

You only have control over three things in your life-the thoughts you think, the images you visualize, & the actions you take.
~Jack Canfield

We cannot say it enough, experiencing an occasional funk is completely normal. It's not fun, but it *is* normal. Unfortunately, that's just life.

From time to time you are going to experience these kinds of emotions. And although you have no control over their arrival, your response to these emotions is one hundred percent controlled by you. The take-home message here is this: you are in control of your thoughts, attitudes, and choices.

Not only are you in control of exercising your right to choose, you also get to determine the outcome. Here are the two possible outcomes you may choose between:

Outcome #1: Become Stronger
Outcome #2: Become Weaker

It appears to be a no-brainer, but all too often we inadvertently choose Outcome #2. This happens because we give in to the negative emotions and allow them to dictate our actions. This could be turning to food or trying to medicate ourselves some other way—wasting time, procrastinating, or tuning things out hoping for time to pass quickly.

On the other hand, if we choose Outcome #1, we can take advantage of the times we are in a funk by engaging in a productive activity or mindset. Not only will it minimize the length of our funk days but it will have positive impact down the road.

These are our two choices. When we choose Outcome #1 we are growing in character, setting ourselves up for success, and developing steady and stable lives. Outcome #2, on the other hand, will only keep us living in a constant state of chaos and instability. We can avoid living like that. Our life can be better.

Keep calm and carry on.

Understand Some Days Will Be Tough

Lara

When we were working on this book I came across an old blog post I had written around the holidays a couple years back. I thought some of you might be able to relate:

Some days, no matter what or how much I eat, I still feel unsatisfied. Then, as I frantically try to find a hidden candy stash, I scream inside, "What are you doing? Stop eating! Why are you STILL eating?!"

Even though my weight only fluctuates five to ten pounds, I still have days when I fall off the deep end. Thinking it will make me feel better, I eat everything in sight, when in fact it only makes me feel worse and causes me to eat more. I basically give up on myself and hope tomorrow is a better day, which usually isn't any better because I wake up feeling horrible due to a food hangover!

I'll be honest; I don't have a glorious ending to this post. I'm just writing to say no matter what size or weight you are, some days are just tough. Even in the most perfect circumstances, peace with food will be challenging from time to time.

Speaking of which, I don't know about you, but the holiday goodies are making this "eating stuff" even more difficult. I'm trying to sample in moderation, but again…trying to be real with you here…it is a struggle, and some days I just want to give up.

Confession: Right before I sat down to write this post, I had intentions of ending my horrible eating day with a glass of milk and cookies. I just happened to text my sis, my accountability partner, and she said she was at the gym. Hearing from her is what it took to "snap out of it." Instead, I've opted to write you and save myself the extra calories and disappointment I would have felt in ten minutes. Thank you, sis, and to my readers, for detouring my thoughts so my day could end better than expected! You are NEVER alone.

Find a Posse Partner

Surround yourself with only people who are going to lift you higher.
~Oprah Winfrey

Lara

Think of the qualities that make a good friendship. I envision two gal pals, like Gayle King and Oprah. I imagine them chatting it up as they talk about the details of their day. One of them curled up with her feet in the couch while the other sinks into a comfy chair, laughing hysterically about an embarrassing moment from the lunch hour. It is obvious there is no topic that goes off-limits in their relationship. I don't know about you, but I think that defines a good friendship!

For as long as I can remember I have tried losing weight. During my pre-kid days, I was always trying different weight loss tactics to shed those last several pounds. When I had my first baby, it became even more of a challenge. I tried all the diets and exercise plans that I could, but I wasn't having success. I was never tenacious enough to stick it out on my own. I had debated for years about taking a leap of faith and asking someone to hold me accountable and be my *Posse Partner*. I pushed it off because it was frightening to reach out for help in this way.

I knew if I decided to quit my diet no one would ever know. In reality, I was setting myself up for failure before I ever started! And although asking someone to help was scary, it would ultimately determine how serious I was about changing. I eventually found the courage and, believe it or not, it wasn't until I had a Posse Partner that I finally had some success with my weight loss!

Finding the right person to share your journey with is important. My Posse Partner has changed over the years. At one time it was my sister, and although we lived far apart, I shared my weigh-in number with her every week. We couldn't work out together, but texted or called with how things were going (good or bad).

In recent years, Robynn has been the one I confide in. I know that even if I admit I have eaten half a bag of cookies or weighed myself ten times in one day, she will still care about me. Like any Posse Partner should, she will listen. We will talk through what happened so I can use my experience as a meaningful lesson for the future. We spend countless hours discussing our struggles and victories when it comes to losing weight. Some days start with, "I had a breakthrough!" while other days begin somberly with, "I need a pep talk."

Like Oprah and Gayle, you need to find someone you can be transparent and real with. Whatever crazy things you think or do, your Posse Partner won't judge but will continue to encourage.

Even better, find someone who has been successful doing what you are trying to do—lose weight and do it with peace. Most likely they will be thrilled to help, and you won't have to reinvent the wheel. You can use their experience and can learn from their successes and failures.

We like what Jeff Olson, author of *The Slight Edge,* says:

Whatever goals you aspire to, seek out people who have achieved the same or very similar goals or who are well along that path, and go camp on their doorsteps or do whatever you can to associate with them, emulate them, and let their grasp, understanding, and mastery of the subject rub off on you.[3]

Good advice.

If there is a habit you can't kick, reach out to a friend or support group and ask them for help. Assemble your posse. It not only will strengthen your relationship, but will have positive results toward achieving your goal.

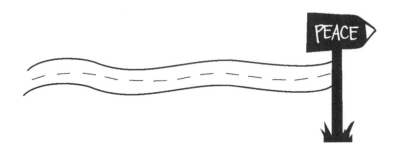

G. Gas Station
How and Where You Can Fuel-Up—What can you do/whom can you rely on to stay motivated?

- _____
- _____
- _____
- _____
- _____
- _____

Lara: Call Robynn! And if she doesn't answer, I crank up some music, put on my running shoes, and find something to accomplish before the end of the day.

Robynn: I pray, read my Bible, listen to inspiring music and talks on DVD's. Lara and I talk often, which also charges my batteries. Exercise also gives me a big boost and energizes me physically and mentally.

Get Help from God

There are many things that are essential to arriving at true peace of mind, and one of the most important is faith, which cannot be acquired without prayer.
~John Wooden

Robynn

In the process of writing this book, Lara installed tile in her house. In case you didn't know, she loves to complete do-it-yourself projects. She is constantly taking on a new venture such as installing countertops and putting up trim, and she's even hung kitchen cabinets by herself! Impressive, I know.

During the course of installing tile, she secured underlayment to the floor where she literally used thousands of nails. That is a lot of nails! That number sounds even more massive when you're the one doing the work.

To make the project a thousand times easier, Lara didn't use a hammer, she used a nail gun. Had she tried to complete the project using only a hammer, chances are she would have lost energy and motivation, likely causing the floor to remain unfinished to this day.

When I think of that hammer and nail gun, I think of the journey Lara and I have taken to find peace with food. We've been at it for a while and, had we taken the hammer approach, I'm quite certain we would have given up a long time ago. We wouldn't have had the power to complete the task on our own. Instead, we needed a *nail gun.*

That's why we enlisted help from God. By doing so we tapped into a power source much greater than our own. We share this with you because we want to give you an honest and accurate picture of how we have reached that incredible place known as peace with food. For us, it is a major piece of the puzzle and we would be remiss to not share the truth about a significant part of how we got to where we are.

If you've been taking the hammer approach and are about to run out of power, you may want to reach for the *nail gun.* I am quite certain that once you make the switch, you will never go back.

Be Practical

Lara

As I cleaned up the mess in the kitchen, a single chocolate chip dropped out of its bag. Time stood still as it hit the counter, landing as if it were staring right at me. "What is one chocolate chip?" I thought to myself. "But if I eat it, I'll blow it because I'm on a no-sweets diet." I didn't want to lose control, but it kept gawking at me, reminding me I had been sweet-deprived for days. Well guess what? I ate it. So then what? I blew it. I said, "Forget it!" and I porked out the rest of the night.

Peace with food deals with real life, not some pie-in-the-sky fantasy world that promises miraculous results in a few short days. Considering this, you need to be realistic. The following are some of the realities in the pursuit of reaching your healthy weight and a life of tranquility.

- **Shoot for progress, not perfection.** We are not shooting for perfection (because it doesn't exist) but for consistency and continual improvement. We would consider this a success. Just don't stop there!
- **Sacrifice is inevitable.** You have probably heard the saying "No pain, no gain." We don't subscribe to extreme methods. However, if you want to get to your healthy weight, you may have to tell yourself, "No" from time to time. As we've already said, when it comes to eating: You can eat whatever you want, as long as it brings you peace.
- **You have to start where you are.** Yes, this sounds obvious, but many people are so distraught by how much they weigh, it causes them to postpone this crucial choice to change their life. Which leads us to…
- **You don't have forever.** Every day you put off walking in peace is yet another day you will never get back.

Living a life of happiness will require an understanding that perfection is impossible. Instead, strive for continual progress.

Take One Small Step

In order to make dreams come into reality, it takes an awful
lot of determination, dedication, self-discipline, and effort.
~Jesse Owens

Grinding gears, smoke coming from under the hood, and our dads shaking their heads and chuckling at our attempt to help on the farm. That is the familiar scene we both experienced as farm girls. There we stood, sweat dripping down our faces as we killed the engine, something we often experienced for the nth time. Hey, at least we get an "A" for effort.

Learning to drive with a stick shift takes practice. As with any skill you wish to acquire, there is a learning curve. Living at peace is no different.

Beginning this journey will give you a taste of freedom and control like you've never experienced. Unfortunately it isn't mastered right away and requires developing skills, which takes time. But like a turkey that cooks "slow and low" on Thanksgiving Day, it is well worth the wait when you take that first bite. It's like any character trait you are attempting to develop.

Let's say you are an extremely impatient person, but you make a commitment to develop patience. You can't expect perfection by tomorrow, but by chipping away at the goal, day by day, you will begin to see progress. Even when you feel this trait has been mastered, you may struggle from time to time. However, you will find the failures are fewer than when you first started.

It may surprise you when we say it took years to identify what peace with food was and to learn to walk it out. The good news for you is that you don't have to spend years experimenting. We've already done that for you. Instead, you can hit the ground running and use our mistakes, successes, and lessons to your advantage.

Along the way there will be discoveries for you to make regarding what brings you peace. Although we won't give you a set of strict rules, we can help steer you in the right direction. So keep your hands on the wheel and make the commitment to hang in there. Even when the road gets bumpy, refusing to quit will get you to your destination while you take the ride of your life!

Chapter 5 Take-Home Messages

✓Give yourself grace to be who you are. Enjoy your unique self and don't try to fit into someone else's mold. Do what works best for you.

✓You are valuable. Period. You have the choice to live purposefully or purposelessly.

✓To get the biggest bang for your buck, prioritize and determine what people and activities will get the most amount of your time.

✓Winning in peace with food isn't about the quick fix. It's about gaining the skill that will help you be more precise.

✓Hit the reset button by making a choice.

✓You are who you hang around with. Assess the role your family and friends play in your eating habits.

✓Experiencing the funk is normal to life. Your response will determine whether your outcome is positive or negative.

✓You are in control of your thoughts, attitudes, and choices.

✓To jumpstart your posse, begin working through the discussion guide in the back of this book.

✓Tap into a power source much greater than your own by getting help from above.

✓Living in happiness will require an understanding that perfection is impossible. Instead, strive for continual progress.

✓Although beginning this journey will give you a taste of freedom and control, it isn't mastered right away and requires developing skills, which takes time.

CHAPTER

6

Weight

Be Smart with the Scale

The choice to lead an ordinary life is no longer an option.
~Spider-Man

Lara

I had decided one of my experiments for this book would be taking a break from weighing in on my scale. At the time, my family and I were in the middle of relocating, so this was a perfect time to throw the scale in a moving box and hide it for a few months to keep me from changing my mind.

During the course of our move, we stayed with various family and friends. As I woke up one morning from an overnight stay, for whatever reason, I wasn't thinking very rationally. I had been feeling good (thin) and saw a scale in the bathroom. Surely it wouldn't hurt to take a peek at my current weight since I hadn't weighed myself for weeks. *What was I thinking?!* Not only was I going to weigh in on a completely different scale, which may or may not be accurate, I was also weighing in at a different time of day, under different circumstances.

As I stepped on the scale, I immediately went from feeling as light as a feather to as heavy as a dump truck. Sure enough, it showed a weight gain of a few pounds, and I panicked! What had I done?

At that point, it was war. I was bound and determined to prove to myself that this scale was wrong. I made it my mission to find my hidden scale. Thankfully, I knew our moving boxes were in an old building not far from where we were staying, so the hunt began instantly. I'm not even sure what I did with my kids at that point, because all I could think about was finding that scale. A few numbers on a different scale had unleashed a monster!

Sprawled out like an action figure, I attempted a Spider-Man move with my left foot propped on an old stove, my right foot on some plastic storage tubs, and my body twisted under a rolled up piece of carpet that had been wedged to hang in the air. I could see "the box." With sweat rolling down my face, I wasn't going to let anything come between me and that cardboard container. It held my most precious piece of evidence to verify that the number on the scale that morning was wrong.

It is amazing the extreme measures we go through in order to prove a point, because to this day, the final seconds leading up to getting "the box" are still a blur. Regardless, I remember the satisfaction I felt when I held that old, worn scale in my hands. I gained my composure and...*gulp*...stripped down to nothing (which we all know is essential in getting the most accurate reading!)...as I stood on my scale waiting patiently for the dotted line to finally flash my anticipated number.

After what seemed like eternity—*whew!*—the scale showed that I hadn't gained a pound since my last weigh-in several weeks prior. What a relief, but what a nightmare I had experienced in the last hour.

It is frightening how quickly we can slip into our insane cycle. Had I only done the right thing, I would never have weighed in on a different scale and set myself up to fail. It not only caused stress but made me second guess myself, regardless of the fact I'd been feeling and eating great.

My advice after this catastrophe is to avoid making rash decisions when it comes to weighing in, and don't convince yourself you can mimic Spider-Man when desperately trying to reach for something! I was sore for days... *Yikes!*

Decide What You Really Want

There is one quality which one must possess to win, and that is the definiteness of purpose, the knowledge of what one wants, and a burning desire to possess it.
~Napoleon Hill.

Robynn

Years ago, I bought myself a pair of white dress shorts as my motivator. These shorts were two sizes smaller than what I was currently wearing, and fitting into them was what I considered the ultimate goal. As I continued to lose weight, which ended up being more than initially planned, I began comfortably fitting into the next size down, but my white shorts were still a bit too tight.

Unfortunately, because I was so transfixed on those silly shorts and have tendencies of an all-or-nothing mindset, I was unable to enjoy all the other clothes I would have dreamed to wear back in the day! I even loved the way I looked, but couldn't enjoy my successes until I achieved the ultimate one—fitting loosely in those white shorts.

Wow, those shorts taught me a great lesson. And who knows, I may keep them around for a very long time as a reminder to never lose sight of what I really want.

As you begin to ponder what you really want, initially you may think it is having a healthy and fit body or being a certain number on the scale. It's easy to get caught up in things that aren't really all that important, while overlooking the true yearning of our hearts. From experience, we can tell you: don't miss the forest for the trees.

There is a quote that says, "There are many things in life that will catch your eye, but only a few will catch your heart...pursue those."

If a skinny model captured your eye with her body when, really, your heart has the desire to feel alive, healthy, and fully present in life, then it is time to sit yourself down. Take the time to have a good heart-to-heart with yourself and answer this question: What is it that *you* really want?

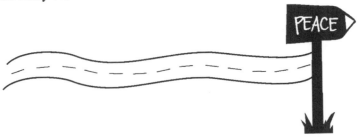

H. Reflection in the Window

What You Want—What is it that you really want regarding your body and your weight?

- _____
- _____
- _____
- _____
- _____
- _____
- _____

Lara: I want to be happy based on how I look in the mirror and how I feel physically, not based on the number on the scale. When my weight fluctuates, I tend to change my emotions because of the number on the scale. Because of this, I avoid weighing in on a daily basis. It effects my feelings too much—usually in a negative way—and often results in my turning to food.

Robynn: First and foremost I want to live in peace. For me, the best way to do that is by being fit and consistently staying in my realistic weight range even during the "off" times such as vacations or holidays.

Find Your Optimal Weight Zone

In baseball, my theory is to strive for consistency, not to worry about the numbers. If you dwell on statistics you get shortsighted, if you aim for consistency, the numbers will be there at the end.
~Tom Seaver, Baseball Hall-of-Famer

Being Kansans, we are accustomed to people commenting to us about *The Wizard of Oz*. In fact, if we meet you for the first time and you are at least three states removed from Kansas, the likelihood of your mentioning this iconic movie increases dramatically. Ask any Kansan and they will probably agree.

In *The Wizard of Oz*, the Land of Oz represents a desirable and idyllic place. There is a similar Land of Oz in peace with food. We call it your Optimal Weight Zone. This zone is the weight range you feel is best for you.

If you have watched Bobby Flay in the kitchen or an Olympic gold medalist in competition, you know how flawless these people appear as they do what they do best (and the rest of us admire). What's common among such people is they are in their zone as they effortlessly perform their skill.

You may have experienced being "in the zone" in some area of your life. Maybe it was athletics, a performance, or an activity where you found yourself in this wonderfully, exhilarating experience. The zone is where things click—an uncanny and maybe even surreal ease that sends you soaring.

Your body has a zone concerning its weight range. Your optimal weight zone is where:

- You physically and psychologically feel your best.
- You have peace.
- Your body naturally finds the best fit for the predetermined physical attributes you've been given—your physical makeup, frame, musculature, and metabolism.

Determining your zone would be nice if someone could just tell you, but it's not that easy. It will take time to find out exactly what that range is, but you can use some of the following tools as guidelines. We repeat, as guidelines, not as absolutes. For the average person they can get you in the ball park of your zone, but they are not to be taken as infallible and accurate. Use them as estimates, but as we always say, ultimately follow peace.

Two common standards used by physicians and health professionals:

- **BMI**—Body Mass Index (BMI) is a number calculated from a person's weight and height. BMI provides a reliable indicator of body fatness for most people and is used to screen for weight categories that may lead to health problems. (Centers for Disease Control and Prevention)[4]
- **Weight Range**—A list of heights with their corresponding recommended weight. To get a more accurate number, you may want to use the frame size (wrist) calculator.

We strongly advise you to find a weight range (optimal weight zone) and not get focused on just one number. That's because your body is constantly fluctuating in its weight, and becoming obsessed with a number will definitely get you on the insane cycle.

However, in finding your optimal weight zone and maintaining it, you will still be experiencing success even if you're not at your ideal weight. Use these questions to help determine your optimal weight zone:

- What weight range does your dietitian/physician recommend?
- At what weight do you feel the healthiest?
- What weight gives you peace?
- Will the sacrifices made to reach your desired weight exceed the enjoyment of actually being at that weight? If so, you may want to adjust that number. Maybe your goal needs to be ten pounds more than your desired weight to make exercise and eating experiences more enjoyable. Although maybe not ideal, if you look and feel good, the sacrifice of a few extra pounds is definitely something to consider.

One piece of advice we like comes from a Weight Watchers® leader Karen McCoy, who says there is a difference between a weight being attainable and a weight being maintainable. Using this bit of wisdom you may want to make the high end of your weight zone a number that is maintainable and the low end a number that is attainable.

Finding your Land of Oz may take time and experimentation but when you reach it, you'll know. Best of all, once you get there you won't be disappointed by smoke and mirrors. Instead you'll experience a deep sense of peace knowing you are right where you should be.

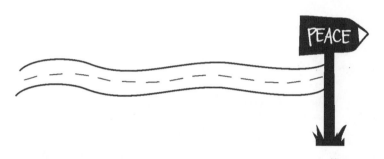

I. Land of Oz
Your Optimal Weight Zone
At what weight do you feel physically and psychologically best?

_____

What weight range does your dietitian/physician recommend?

_____

What weight does your body naturally find the best fit for the predetermined physical attributes you've been given—your physical makeup, frame, musculature and metabolism?

_____

What weight gives you peace?

_____

Lara: I feel the absolute best in the mid to lower end of the healthy range of my BMI.

Being there though, takes extra work to maintain and doesn't allow me to eat as much as I would like. That being said, without much effort, my body seems to naturally stay at the middle, healthy range of my BMI. I don't feel the best at that weight, but I can be more laid back in what I eat and how active I am. I certainly shouldn't feel bad if I am in this range because I am still considered healthy and am able to find the energy to chase my kids!

Robynn: My answer to all the above would be somewhere in the middle of my recommended healthy range of my BMI.

Budget Your Calories

Budget, for many people, is a word that makes them cringe. It's probably because they think it means depriving themselves of what they want most and requires a great deal of self-control. Or maybe they feel inadequate and aren't sure how to create and maintain a budget.

If you can relate to any of the above, relax. A budget can be really rewarding, because a budget—whether you are talking about food, money, or time—is a guideline of how you choose to spend your resources. The beauty of budgeting is getting to call the shots and being in control.

When budgeting a monthly allotment of income, you determine how much to spend within each category—housing, groceries, and clothing. The same applies to eating. Once you calculate the number of calories you will allot yourself each day, you can determine how you will spend those calories.

One skill of budgeting is prioritization. You have to rank what is most important to least important. There will be times that least important items need to go to the wayside to avoid overspending. And don't forget, you can have bad results by overspending money just as you can with overeating calories. The only difference is that eating more calories causes weight gain while overspending puts you in debt.

If you eat out with your coworkers numerous times each week, and the meals are typically high in calories, you may be overspending your calories. If you are serious about getting down to your optimal weight zone, you may have to cut out some of these extra calories by ordering healthier, low calorie meals or eating half of what you would normally order.

Remember, a budget is actually a good thing. It's a gauge of your caloric balance, but gives you the freedom to spend those calories however you choose.

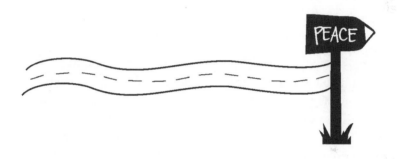

J. The Bank

Budgeting Calories—Are you having a difficult time getting to your optimal weight zone? If so, where are you overspending? Jot down where you are going over budget in your eating.

- _____
- _____
- _____
- _____
- _____

Lara: When I get lazy and don't create a situation where I have closure with what I am eating, I usually end up getting "just one more bite" of something, which turns in to several more bites and ends up being wasted calories.

Robynn: Typically, if I overspend on calories, it's before lunch. My number one temptation may be to keep eating at breakfast which sets me up to overeat the rest of the day. My solution is to get busy and "rip it." If I can make it to lunch without overspending, chances of my staying inbounds the rest of the day are high.

Invest in Peace

You aren't going to find anybody that's going to be successful without making a sacrifice and without perseverance.
~Lou Holtz

What is the price you have to pay to get to your goal? What is the least amount of effort required to get there? What are you willing to invest without sacrificing peace?

Losing weight is a math equation. If you eat more than your body burns, you will gain weight. If you want to lose weight, you need to burn more calories than you consume. If you are content with your weight, you can continue eating as much as you are burning in calories each day.

Calories Consumed + Physical Activity = Your Weight

The same applies to money. Let's use the same paragraph as above but replace a few words. If you spend more than you make, you will go into debt. If you want to be rich, you need to make more than you spend. If you are content with your finances, you can continue spending as much as you are bringing in each day.

Decide how much you are willing to sacrifice. For us, we know we will lose all peace if we expect ourselves to sacrifice birthday cake with our kids or big meals at family get-togethers. Therefore, if we are realistic, we know eating those extra calories will require burning the same amount of calories to avoid a weight gain. Either that or accept the fact we will gain weight, which will take a while to shed if we don't exercise.

It's time for you to have a talk with yourself and determine the price you are willing to pay. This is a choice only you can make. For us, the price changed when we committed to our journey. We no longer were willing to exercise and eat in such a way that would steal our peace, joy, and freedom.

```
Lara: If I know I want to eat a big meal or a
large helping of dessert in the evening, I
make a point to get more exercise throughout
the day. By doing so, it makes the dessert
even more enjoyable because I know my
activities helped offset my larger calorie
consumption.
```

Determine Your Caloric Intake

Once you've determined the price you are willing to pay, it may be beneficial to learn the number of calories needed to reach your goal weight. There are an abundance of resources to help including the USDA's *My Plate* recommendation, which replaced the food pyramid most of us grew up with. Another option is a plan such as Weight Watchers®.

The amount of information out there can be overwhelming. As we state throughout this book, there is no one-size-fits-all plan, so you will need to invest in discovering what works best for you.

One tool we have found helpful is a body weight/calorie simulator that calculates the daily consumption of calories needed to reach your weight loss goal. You simply input your current weight, goal weight, goal date, and a few other items. One such simulator can be found on the National Institute of Health's website.

Focus on Your Progress with the Scale

During the peace with food process you will occasionally hit a wall. This usually occurs when the scale won't budge. People also feel this way when they've lost a lot of weight, but still have a lot left to lose.

Say your starting weight was 220 pounds and you are now at 180 pounds. Back at your starting weight you would have been ecstatic to be in the 180's but now your goal is to reach the 150's and the scale won't budge. Doubt starts creeping in your mind and you wonder if this concept really works. You think you should throw in the towel and convince yourself it can't be done.

In that moment, use your voice of reason. Instead of stressing over a stubborn couple of pounds, focus on how far you've come. Close your eyes and remember what life was like at 220 pounds and how losing forty pounds seemed so unattainable at the time. It's crazy how quickly we fail to appreciate our progress after time has lapsed. As soon as the newness of our situation wears off, we start beating ourselves up. Sounds like another insane cycle.

Seriously, you've lost forty pounds my friend! Focus on where you've come from, not where you are currently stuck!

When you find yourself feeling frustrated or panicked, use your voice of reason. Take a deep breath and remind yourself of your progress to date. Even if it isn't in pounds, you can still give yourself a pat on the back for the character and commitment to walk this journey out. That alone, is a great improvement. Don't underestimate the value in that.

Chapter 6 Take-Home Messages

✓ Don't make rash decisions when it comes to weighing in on the scale.

✓ What is the true desire of your heart regarding your body, self-esteem, and what you really want out of life?

✓ Your Land of Oz is your optimal weight zone.

✓ A food budget allows you to set a guideline of how you will spend your calories.

✓ What are you willing to invest without sacrificing peace?

✓ An online body weight/calorie simulator may be a helpful tool in determining how many calories you need to consume daily.

✓ Focus on how far you've come instead of how far you have left to go.

Exercise Won't Solve All Your Problems

Robynn

For years I stared down at those last ten to fifteen unwanted pounds that refused to come off. I was constantly looking for the elixir that would help melt those pounds away. Maybe it was a new diet, maybe it was a new exercise program. I just knew there was something out there that would help me achieve my objective.

Being a runner, when the idea of a marathon popped into my brain, I was sure I had the answer to my weight loss dilemma. So that's exactly what I did, I began training for a marathon. And although it wasn't purely for weight loss, it certainly was an incentive. After four months of logging my training hours, I actually ended up gaining six pounds. Yes, six pounds! And the second time around wasn't much better—even though I didn't gain weight, I didn't lose much either! The point is, it is so easy to think a marathon, a new diet, or new workout is going to be your answer. I call this the marathon myth, and although these things aren't bad, *per se*, they aren't a magic bullet. They are just a means, not the end. These things, by themselves, will not bring you peace because they are external and when it comes to peace, remember, it's an inside job, baby!

Use a Variety of Exercise Routines

Robynn

A country road.

On a summer morning.

At the crack of dawn.

With a dog named Paws.

This is where I got hooked on running. It all began when I was a teenager getting in shape for the sport I loved—basketball. Little did I know the hold it would have on me, resulting in a lifetime of commitment and devotion.

I'm not sure how it snagged me. It was a combination of things. The way it made me feel. The sight of a calming countryside. The smell of fresh air and fresh-cut hay. The stillness that allowed my mind to ponder and pray.

Or maybe it was running past my Aunt Gladys's house a mile down the road from mine. She would step out the screen door onto her porch and call out to me as I was running by. "Robby, can you stop for breakfast?" I would answer back, "On my way back, when I finish."

After my run, I would stop by her house, and we would visit in her kitchen over fresh fruit and toast as the morning breeze blew through the open windows and screen door.

I think it is due to all of these reasons that running is the exercise version of my comfort food. I love it.

And although I love it, it's more about the experience than just the activity of burning calories and working the heart. For that reason, I don't like running outside when it's cold, rainy, or windy. I want to feel the warm air on my skin while the birds and insects are chirping around me. Running on a still day brings me happiness. So for me, outdoor running occurs in the spring, summer, and fall, but not in the winter. My goal during these warmer months is to run five to six times a week.

However, I like to switch it up in the winter. The following is a sample of the activities that I either do now or have done in the past that help keep me in the game and give me peace during that time of the year:

- **From November to April**: Run on the treadmill while watching an inspirational talk on television.
- **For one month—30-Day Shred**: A workout DVD by Jillian Michaels. It is only 20 minutes, and I can do that!
- **For one month—21-Day Fix**: A DVD series, by Autumn Calabrese. It is only 30 minutes, and the workouts do a variety of exercises that include using light weights working the arms, legs, core, and other muscles. I really enjoy these workouts, as time seems to fly by when doing them. They have been a great tool to help tone my body.
- **For two months—Insanity**: This DVD series by Shaun T. gets me in incredible shape. Most workouts are over forty minutes; however, when I've worked hard for thirty minutes I'm finished.
- **For two months—Pilates**: A form of exercise that focuses on flexibility and core strength (strength in the abdomen and back). For me, the benefits have been a leaner, stronger, and more flexible body.

These workouts will get me through the doldrums of the winter months from November to March. By then I'm itching to get back outside to run or walk.

As I've said, I like to change it up. I do this more to deal with the boredom issue than to comply with the latest findings of fitness experts.

That may not be the case for you. Maybe you want to run three miles, five days a week, all year long. Then do it. Even though you can get the best results by changing things up, the goal is keeping you in the game and following peace. On the other hand, you may be wired to crave intense workouts and physically demanding activities. Whatever it is, you can't go wrong if it brings you peace.

When trying to find your favorite physical activity, don't dismiss things such as gardening, cleaning, and physically demanding work like construction or farming.

Try things you've never done, but that sound interesting and appealing. Join a spinning class, a martial arts class, or a biking/running/walking club. Sign up for intramurals on a city recreation team. Go play in the backyard with your kids. Spend time visiting with your friends while walking (instead of drinking coffee and eating donuts).

During the summer, when my kids were smaller, my family would bike to the swimming pool multiple times a week—yet another way we worked exercise into our life.

I used to think that, in order to lose weight, I had to work out like a crazy woman. Don't get me wrong. There are times I love to work out with that level of intensity, but not all the time. There are periods when I just want to be active, but not intense. I listen to my body and go with it. Give yourself the freedom to do what works best for you. If you're not there, then don't force it. Don't feel pressure to join your friends who are training for a marathon or working out at the hottest gym, especially if you have already found something you love to do.

Here are some other things I've tried that may be of interest to you:

- **Membership at a Fitness Center or Gym**: At times I get a membership at Rehabilitation and Fitness Center during the winter. It allows me to walk, run, lift weights, or bike. I'm grateful for this place because it was where I was able to drop my excess sixty plus pounds after my last baby.
- **CrossFit®**: A conditioning program used by many police academies, fire departments, military personal, elite athletes, as well as those who are first-time exercisers. It emphasizes a broad range of exercises. The daily workouts are intense and varied; however, many of them are relatively short. CrossFit® is growing in

popularity, and chances are, you have a CrossFit® gym near you. I have been amazed to see people who have never been active, become fitness buffs due to CrossFit®. This is possible because in CrossFit® you are competing against yourself and working at your own level. CrossFit® helped me get in excellent shape. I only did it for a few months during the winter. I stopped because I was unable to do many of the lifts due to a back injury, and I wanted to be able to exercise outdoors during the summer. My husband Scott, a former weightlifter, does CrossFit® at home by accessing workouts on the Internet. If you are looking for camaraderie in exercising, want to switch things up daily, are looking for a challenge, or want to increase your strength, this approach may be exactly what you are looking for.

- **High-Intensity Interval Training (HIIT)**: After reading many articles on the benefits of HIIT, I was finally convinced when I read, "Interval workouts burn calories like lighter fluid." I followed a plan my fitness center had posted. I had such great results from doing HIIT that people would often ask me what I was doing. Here it is below:

HIIT TRAINING SCHEDULE

WEEK	MAX EFFORT	REST	REPS
1	1 MIN	2 MIN	5
2	1 MIN	90 SEC	6
3	1 MIN	1 MIN	8
4	1 MIN	1 MIN	10
5	75 SEC	1 MIN	10
6	90 SEC	1 MIN	10

Warm up five minutes before HIIT with a light jog. I always go for thirty minutes and use whatever time is left for easy jogging.

You can use the following as cheat sheets when you are on the treadmill so you don't have to try to remember when you are supposed to be going at your max effort and when you are supposed to be walking.

WEEK 2—Begin with a jog until 5:00 MIN	
Begin running at max effort:	Begin walking at:
5:00 MIN	6:00 MIN
7:30 MIN	8:30 MIN
10:00 MIN	11:00 MIN
12:30 MIN	13:30 MIN
15:00 MIN	16:00 MIN
17:30 MIN	18:30-20:00 MIN
Jog until 30:00 MIN	

WEEK 5—Begin with a jog until 5:00 MIN	
Begin running at max effort:	Begin walking at:
5:00 MIN	6:15 MIN
7:15 MIN	8:30 MIN
9:30 MIN	10:45 MIN
11:45 MIN	13:00 MIN
14:00 MIN	15:15 MIN
16:15 MIN	17:30 MIN
18:30 MIN	19:45 MIN
20:45 MIN	22:00 MIN
23:00 MIN	24:15 MIN
25:15 MIN	26:30-27:30 MIN
Jog until 30:00 MIN	

WEEK 6—Begin with a jog until 2:30 MIN	
Begin running at max effort:	Begin walking at:
2:30 MIN	4:00 MIN
5:00 MIN	6:30 MIN
7:30 MIN	9:00 MIN
10:00 MIN	11:30 MIN
12:30 MIN	14:00 MIN
15:00 MIN	16:30 MIN
17:30 MIN	19:00 MIN
20:00 MIN	21:30 MIN
22:30 MIN	24:00 MIN
25:00 MIN	26:30-27:30 MIN
Jog until 30:00 MIN	

Also, don't disregard the opportunities presented in your everyday life. As an all-or-nothing person, I always turned up my nose at walking. However, after an injury I had no choice, so I started walking the same distance as I would typically run, and I had great results. The take-home message: Use the resources you have.

Non-Traditional Exercise

Lara

When people hear the words *workout* or *exercise,* they usually think of running, going to the gym, playing a sport, or training for a marathon. Believe it or not, none of those things sound appealing to me, at least at this time in my life. I still burn calories, but my workout routine doesn't consist of the conventional types of exercise.

My typical day is filled with chasing kids, changing diapers, picking up the house, and running my home business. In addition to those tasks, my favorite hobby is decorating and constantly changing the interior of our home. Call me crazy, but most weeks include my rearranging furniture in a room (by myself), starting a new project such as tearing out flooring, hanging trim, or painting, and fixing broken appliances or furniture around the house. Doing that type of work really fuels me. I love it.

While Robynn and I were trying to figure out this whole peace with food thing, we talked a lot about the need to exercise. Poor Robynn...I'm sure every time we discussed it, I was a broken record. I would repeatedly tell her I needed to start running on my treadmill because it was the only way I felt I could exercise. And sure enough, after a few weeks of dragging myself to the basement and logging twenty minutes on the treadmill, I lost motivation. Months later I'd muster up the energy to try it again, with the same result of boredom. I mean seriously, there is no fun when you are running in place while staring at an ugly, concrete wall! Being a decorating addict, you can only imagine how much I wanted to get off that stinkin' machine and give those dreadful walls a complete makeover!

When I complained about my exercise struggle, Robynn suggested I was probably underestimating the number of calories I was burning doing housework. I would chuckle, because if I told people my exercise was "being active around the house" they would probably write it off as an excuse, since it doesn't fall into the traditional way of keeping fit.

> Work out but don't freak out if it doesn't fall under the traditional ways to exercise. Stay active by doing things you enjoy.

It wasn't until Robynn bought me a Fitbit® that my whole perspective changed. (Side note, this is how you define a true friend: Someone who gives you an activity tracker right after having baby number three, and tells you it *isn't* because you need to lose weight. Ha!). After wearing it for several weeks of doing my normal daily routine, she proved to be right. I was indeed burning a lot of calories by doing what I love most: house projects! I remember one day while deep cleaning and laying grout for our new tiled floor, my activity tracker buzzed before noon, alerting me I had already walked five miles. To boot, that afternoon some girlfriends and I attended a street walk event. By the end of the day it said I had gone 9.44 miles/20,980 steps and burned 3,243 calories! Is that not crazy?! And it hadn't involved one minute on a treadmill!

Today if you were to ask me if I exercise, I would confidently respond by telling you I walk about five miles a day. I would also say, "You don't have to live at the gym to have peace." In fact, the thought of walking on a treadmill or lifting weights is the furthest thing from giving me peace at this time of my life.

I continue to wear my activity tracker and do my very best to get in five miles a day. Rarely do I actually go outside and hit a trail to walk. I can typically accomplish this by doing household tasks all day long. It feels good that, by the end of the day, I am able to accomplish projects I enjoyed and also get several miles of exercise in.

As I have said before, you need to be the authority. We think if we are not doing things like everyone else, it won't work, or we are failing. This is not true. I wasn't doing traditional exercise, but my activity tracker proves that what I do works the same as if I'd walked five miles on a treadmill. For more ideas, here are some other non-traditional ways to exercise:

- **Walking in Place**: My sister lost ten pounds by walking in her living room. Yes, that's right, just walking in place in front of the television!
- **Timed Task**: Growing up, I absolutely hated timed tests in school. Now that I am older, I've found a timed test that I benefit from and somewhat enjoy. After putting my shoes on—to get myself moving—I time myself when needing to complete tasks. I know I can clean off the kitchen counters and unload/reload the dishwasher in four minutes and fifty-four seconds! If I am dreading going through the junk piles of mail and randomness, I set the timer for five minutes and see if I can get through everything before the timer buzzes. Sometimes I send a picture text to my posse or ask my kids to challenge me on tasks for moral support and accountability to finish. They hold the timer and give me the countdown. I literally run through the house in order to beat the clock. If I don't finish it in time, I set the timer again. This not only gets my heart rate up, but it helps me be more efficient with my time.

I am a strong believer in staying active by doing things you enjoy. Maybe you love to shop and you are underestimating the amount of calories you burn by walking around the mall. If you do something that doesn't fall in the traditional way of exercising, consider getting an activity tracker so you can get a better idea of how many calories you are actually burning.

Find an Exercise That Will Motivate

Regarding exercise, we have a litmus test we use for determining what's in and what's out. We also use this litmus test in other areas of our journey, and with life in general.

The litmus test consists of two criteria—questions we ask ourselves:

- Does it keep me in the game?
- Does it give peace?

Use these two questions to help you determine what exercise works best for you.

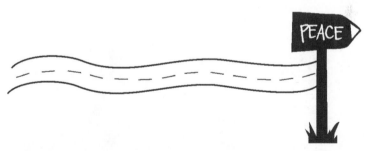

K. The Bike/Running Path
Exercise—What physical activities keep you in the game? What are your exercise preferences?

- _____
- _____
- _____
- _____
- _____

Lara: In terms of traditional exercise, I really don't do much, but I am far from inactive. Instead, I like to do yard work, fix fences (remember I live on a farm!), and do-it-yourself projects that have me doing demo work, moving furniture, redoing floors, and painting.

Robynn: Run and walk in the warm months. Mix it up with interval training in the cold months.

Chapter 7 Take-Home Messages

✓Don't rely on traditional exercise alone to be the magic bullet.

✓Your choice of exercise should keep you in the game and bring you happiness. This may require changing your routine throughout the year.

✓You don't have to live at the gym to have peace. Be creative with ways to stay active and burn calories.

✓When choosing your exercise, figure out what will keep you in the game and what will bring you peace.

CHAPTER

8

Food (A)

Counting Calories on a Twinkie Diet

"Twinkie diet helps nutrition professor lose 27 pounds."

"Twinkies. Nutty bars. Powdered donuts." That is how the CNN article entitled, *"Twinkie diet helps nutrition professor lose 27 pounds"* began.[5]

It details how Kansas State University human nutrition professor, Mark Haub, lost twenty-seven pounds in ten weeks back in 2010 as he conducted his own research on the effects of reducing calories, while consuming sugary foods. His objective was to show it is calories that count, not the nutritional value of the food.

So Haub reduced his calories from 2,600 to 1,800 and consumed convenience store sugary snacks as well as Doritos every three hours.

Here's the results at the end of ten weeks:

	Pre-Twinkie Diet	Post-Twinkie Diet
Weight	201	174
BMI	28.9	24.8
LDL (Bad Cholesterol)		Down 20%
HDL (Good Cholesterol)		Up 20%
Triglycerides (A Form of Fat)		Down 39%
Body Fat	33.4	24.9

We are not telling you to go on a *Twinkie Diet,* however, you may want to consider reaching your optimal weight zone by reducing the calories you consume rather than limiting yourself to eat only certain foods. It may be that eating what you love, using wisdom and moderation, can actually help you lose the extra weight. Allowing yourself foods that you enjoy will also increase your peace by truckloads!

Eat What You Want

As we shared earlier, peace with food is found through allowing yourself to eat whatever you want, as long as it brings you peace. We realize this is a bold statement, so let us explain further.

For years we tried to eat what everyone told us to eat. We did our best to conform to and comply with their rules, but it never brought us freedom and happiness. When we began our journey, however, we took a different approach—that of a scientist. With this mindset, we didn't try to manipulate the results, but instead we were open-minded and unbiased about the outcome.

That was our approach. We just wanted to experiment to see what really worked.

So, in the spirit of experimentation, and using the resources we had, we set off, clueless as to what we would discover.

Feeling so deprived of the foods we loved, we gave ourselves permission to experiment with eating the foods we loved most. And when we did, we were shocked (in a good way) to see our peace level go up. It was unbelievable because we were breaking all the diet rules, yet the joy we experienced was through the roof. Although we allowed ourselves to eat whatever we wanted, we learned early on that if we wanted this level to stay high, we couldn't eat as much as we wanted. There were limits. These limits were similar to the lines on a highway. Going over one line can lead you into the ditch and going over the other line into oncoming traffic. Neither scenario is good, so the lesson we learned was this: keep it between the lines.

Yes, initially we were eating what might be considered a lot of junk food, but this was the first time in our lives we were doing it with permission and in moderation. The end result was peace. As we continued to experiment, we eventually realized that we desired to eat healthier foods, not because we had to or because someone was telling us to, but because for the first time in our lives, we actually wanted to! This was a major breakthrough for us.

This experience gave us a power that dieting never could, a power we had never known, because we were choosing healthy eating. It was unbelievable. Now before you think that we are giving you permission to eat anything regardless of the results, remember, our whole mantra is to *follow peace*. Poor health and excessive weight gain don't give lasting happiness, so eating in a way that is detrimental to your health would be a deal breaker. For us, eating "junk food" for a period of time brought satisfaction because it counteracted the effects of extreme deprivation. It allowed us to psychologically uncoil from years of strict dieting and rule following. It was as if we were making up for all those years of dieting, but doing so in moderation and in a way that brought true bliss. Finally, after all the experimentation, this is what we found to be the most effective:

**You can eat whatever you want,
as long as it brings you peace.**

So these days, before we decide to eat something, here are some questions that we will ask ourselves:

- Will eating _____ bring me peace?
- Will the way I will feel after eating _____ bring me peace?
- What quantity of ____ will bring me the most peace?
- If I don't eat _____, will I regret it and then end up eating something else later to try and make up for it?
- Will eating _____ bring me peace or make me feel deprived if I pass it up?

You may be thinking, "There are no foods that give me peace because eating anything causes me to gain weight." We can understand why you would initially think that. But to further explain, read some of our examples.

Lara:
- Eating birthday cake with my kids brings me happiness because I know if I pass up that special moment it will make me feel deprived (trust me, I LOVE cake!) Plus, if I don't eat it, I will have regrets later, resulting in raiding the pantry to make up for it.
- Currently, what brings me peace is allowing myself to eat one or two cookie dough balls and a glass of milk every night. I enjoy indulging in this treat after the kids are asleep in bed, the house is quiet, and I can finally relax and savor what I am eating. It is the most relaxing part of my day. Earlier in the day, if I am tempted to eat other random sweets, I remind myself that my evening snack (and relaxation time) is what I look forward to the most, which helps me

avoid wasting my calories on other
cookies I may be tempted by.
- I am not a huge pop drinker, but when
it comes to pizza, I really love
having it! Typically, pop would be a
waste of my calories, but if I try
drinking water with pizza, I usually
regret it, which means I head back to
the kitchen later that evening trying
to satisfy the desire, even though
the moment has passed. Over time,
I've learned that letting myself
enjoy pop with pizza is what brings
me the most peace and actually saves
me more calories in the long-run
because I'm not trying to make up for
it later!

Robynn:
- Thanks to this journey, I actually
gave up diet pop. In the past, I had
many unsuccessful attempts at kicking
this habit. But with the mantra of
"follow peace," I determined I wasn't
willing to give up one more day lying
in bed with a splitting headache as my
family enjoyed life without me. I
still miss pop from time to time, but
I have greater peace not drinking it
because I no longer have headaches.
- Drinks with calories are a waste of
calories for me. Every once in a
great while I will enjoy a hot cocoa
on a cold wintry day or an ice cold
glass of lemonade on a summer day,
but for the most part, caloric drinks
are an easy way for me to eliminate
unnecessary calories.

It is important to mention what brings you peace today may not bring you peace later. If Lara finds that pop becomes something she *likes* with pizza, but doesn't *love*, then she will switch back to water or make adjustments depending on how she feels at the time. People change. Moods change. Try to avoid doing things because it is routine, and instead be more conscious about asking if your actions are still bringing you peace.

This is what has worked for us. Now it's time to find out what works for you. Remember, you have to know yourself. Know your health and physical condition. Eating junk food may wreak havoc with your current health condition which would result in no peace. If you suffer from celiac disease, you're not going to find peace by disregarding your condition and diving into a plate of pasta. Maybe that would give temporary satisfaction, but its end result would not give peace.

If there are foods you love, but have made off-limits, it may be time to reintroduce those foods and allow yourself to enjoy them in moderation. Keep reading as we continue to give you more tips on how to do that.

Give Yourself a Psychological Release

Lara

I will never forget the conversation Robynn and I had when we stumbled upon the concept of *Psychological Release*. It was a complete breakthrough in our peace with food journey. There I was, sitting on a barstool in her kitchen, explaining how I was following a very strict eating plan and working out, and the scale wouldn't budge. I felt extremely deprived of all my favorite foods, and I had this internal feeling of a brick wall that came between me and the world (food, the scale, etc.). It was an unpleasant sensation that made me feel trapped in my own body.

I went on to explain that whenever I finally let go and allowed myself to eat what I wanted…whatever I was craving…the need was met and the brick wall crumbled. It was a sense of breaking free, as if I gained strength and could start anew.

We define psychological release as a feast. Although this is a good thing, it can be taken out of bounds.

Psychological Release = Feast

Like driving a car down the highway, if you stay between the lines, you are inbounds. If you cross over, you are out of bounds.

Many times a driver will veer over the lines because they are tired or not paying attention. This is what happens when we have an out-of-bounds psychological release. We mindlessly eat to distract ourselves from our true emotions.

When drivers stay between the lines, it is because they are focused and well-rested. When we are attentive and prepared for a successful psychological release, we stay inbounds.

Characteristics of an inbounds psychological release:
- It gives you peace!
- You refuse to waste your calories. Determine what you really want and make a plan to eat it.
- You do not need to eat large quantities of the food you desire simply because you are giving yourself permission to have a psychological release. If you are craving a crispy chicken sandwich, consider the kid-size version.
- You stop eating when you are satisfied.
- You stop eating when you sense the level of peace is diminishing.
- When you are finished, you remove any remaining food.
- You evaluate your performance after the psychological release. Did you stay inbounds? If not, what caused you to go out of the boundaries you have set?

Characteristics of an out-of-bounds psychological release:
- You want to eat even though no specific food sounds appealing. In other words, you have to think hard about what sounds good.
- You waste calories by eating things that don't sound good or eat food just because it's available.
- You binge to escape emotional pain, discomfort, or negative emotions.
- You experience guilt, not peace.

What we don't want is for you to use a psychological release as an excuse to binge and eat everything in your kitchen. Such behavior wouldn't be considered inbounds. Gorging on anything you can get your hands on and being stuffed to the gills doesn't bring peace. Instead, give yourself permission to eat what you have been craving, using the inbounds guidelines, so you can fill the need and move on.

The idea of being permitted to enjoy the foods you love may feel uncomfortable at first. You may have, in all your dieting experiences, never heard of such a thing. Maybe you thought these foods were bad.

Diets are all about getting quick results, and in order to do that, you have to deprive yourself. But we're not in this thing for a few short weeks. We've enlisted for the long haul.

If you make something forbidden it causes you to eat more and want more. Just like children of strict parents: when finally on their own, they tend to overcompensate due to having felt trapped their entire lives.

No one can tell you what your psychological release will look like because it varies with the person, day, and circumstances. Some people can meet a psychological release without overeating, but for others it may cause overindulging. Whether chicken wings or pecan pie is your psychological release, if you feel like a need was met and can walk away satisfied, you have stayed within your preset boundaries. If you felt guilty, unsatisfied, or if you binged, you were out of bounds.

Lara: I don't weigh myself right after a psychological release. I try to wait a day to allow my inflated weight to come down. If I weigh in early, I prepare myself for a weight gain, knowing I ate more than normal.

Robynn: Weighing in after a psychological release is a reality check for me. It helps me get right back on track.

If you are unsure whether it is an inbounds psychological release, ask yourself the following questions:

- Did I stay within the boundaries of eating only what I desired?
- Did I eat within the boundaries of stopping when the food no longer tasted good?
- Did I have peace after eating?

If you can answer "Yes" to all three questions, then you most likely had an inbounds psychological release.

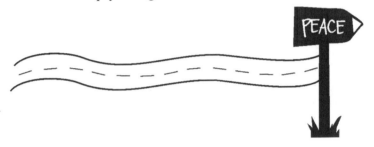

L. Sunset

Psychological Release—When do you need to give yourself permission to just enjoy food and have a Psychological Release?

- _____
- _____
- _____
- _____
- _____
- _____
- _____

Lara: When I feel like I have created a wall between myself and food or when a certain food is calling my name and I know it is a legitimate craving. I am better off eating my craving instead of eating everything else in the house and still feeling unsatisfied. Other than that, I would say your typical "special" events such as date nights and get-togethers.

Robynn: Holidays. Also, from time to time I need to take a break from my healthy eating and just give myself permission to enjoy some of the sweet and salty food I love, but have chosen to eat moderately and only on occasion. A day or two of enjoying these foods usually does the trick and then it is time to get back to my everyday healthy eating habits. This break in the action of healthy eating helps keeps me in the game.

Binge vs. Psychological Release

If a man's wit be wandering, let him study the mathematics.
~Francis Bacon

We can all agree that going on a binge is not a good thing. Now that you have an idea what psychological release is all about, consider this: During the course of a month, add up how many calories you realistically consumed during a recent binge. 500 calories? 1000 calories? Now count up how many calories you consume with an occasional inbounds psychological release. Which one is less?

If you are having an inbounds psychological release, it is not nearly as detrimental to the scale as a throw-in-the-towel binge. When you go on a binge, it is typically accompanied with mindless eating and wasting calories on food you don't love. You are just eating to eat or attempting to fill a void. When we experienced our binges, we generally consumed an additional 1000 calories or more. Considering this, an inbounds psychological release isn't so bad after all. A few extra hundred calories is a small sacrifice if it truly leaves you feeling satisfied and gives you peace.

Allowing yourself to have an inbounds psychological release, when needed, significantly lessens the desire to binge. Do the math. You will lose weight over the course of a year simply by substituting your binging with an inbounds psychological release.

Overindulging Doesn't Bring Peace

One major benefit of peace with food is freedom. After years of dieting, the word *freedom* is sweet music to our ears! Eating whatever you want is the opposite of diets because they restrict what you can and cannot eat. Talk about frustrating! No one wants to live their precious life unable to enjoy the foods they love. Restricting yourself from those foods is simply a recipe for disaster.

Remember you can eat whatever you want, as long as it brings you peace. In this new freedom with food, you are going to have to realize that freedom is not a license to pork out.

The truth is, overindulgence won't give you peace. Maybe you're mistaking it with the temporary high you experience when you're about to binge. But ask yourself if this is a choice you will be happy with later. If tomorrow you will feel regret and despair, then your binge was an out-of-bounds psychological release. It's just that simple.

Eating out of bounds is habit, but many times this habit began due to a variety of reasons. We thought we would share with you the reasons we, and others we know, have developed bad eating habits to help you identify the reasons you may eat out of bounds. Knowing this, you can make efforts to correct bad habits by developing new and improved habits.

Reasons people eat out of bounds:

- Rebelling against a diet. If you have dieted often, your mind and body finally says, "Enough!" and makes up for lost time.
- Attempting to alleviate pain and uncomfortable feelings such as discouragement, boredom, depression, sadness, or hopelessness.
- Not having a plan. If you are traveling with coworkers and don't have a plan, you may end up eating more than you had planned even though you were not very hungry to begin with.

In the rest stop below, identify your reasons for eating out of bounds so you can begin dealing with them. These are the real issues you need to focus on.

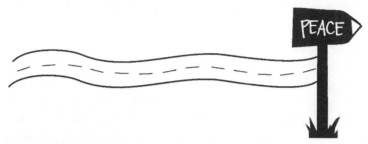

M. Swerve Road Sign

Psychological Release Boundaries—What are your reasons for eating out of bounds? What caused you to eat out of bounds during your last attempt at a psychological release?

- _____
- _____
- _____
- _____
- _____
- _____
- _____

Lara: Not creating a situation where I would have closure with what I was eating.

Robynn: Eating out-of-bounds for me is usually due to an all-or-nothing mindset.

How to Eat Inbounds

A dream doesn't become reality through magic; it takes sweat,
determination and hard work.
~Colin Powell

If your first attempts at a psychological release are failing, remember this: it takes practice. If you've been accustomed to running to food for comfort, entertainment, or relief from uncomfortable feelings, it will take time to develop the good habits needed for an inbounds psychological release. For most people, the skill of staying within the boundaries does not come naturally. Instead, it must be learned. To be successful in any area—money, relationships, time—you will need to learn the appropriate boundaries. The goal here is to hit the bullseye. It won't happen overnight and requires repetition over a period of time before one can expect to master the skill.

Each time you finish a psychological release it is important to evaluate how you did. Assess rather than criticize, condemn, or attack. You are learning a new skill, and that takes time. By assessing and making adjustments, you will begin to make progress. It may be slight, but little by little you'll see your game improve.

Let's imagine a bullseye surrounded by four rings. The bullseye, worth three points, is your target. The next ring is worth two, and so on. Hitting the target will result in an inbounds psychological release.

Use this target evaluation below to help determine your progress.

3—Bullseye! You were inbounds. You did not waste calories and stopped eating when food no longer tasted good. It brought peace before, during, and after the psychological release.

2—You stepped slightly out of bounds, but only a little. Maybe you wasted your calories by eating food you didn't desire. Overall, you came close to hitting the target.

1—You slipped out of bounds by quite a few steps. You not only wasted calories, but you ate beyond feeling full.

0—You completely threw off all restraint and binged. As a result, you wasted a lot calories, ate even though food ceased to give you pleasure, and you lost peace.

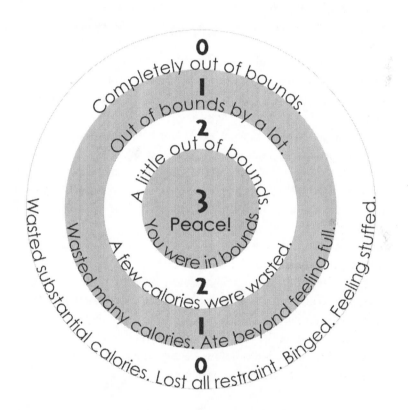

Determine Guilt vs. False Guilt

As we've said, an inbounds psychological release will bring peace and no guilt. However, many people confuse false guilt with true guilt, so we need to address this topic before we continue.

True guilt comes when we do something our conscience tells us is wrong. Guilt is not a bad thing *per se*; it serves as an indicator similar to the red light on the dashboard of a car. It tells us there is something wrong so we know what needs to be fixed. As soon as we take care of the problem, the red light turns green and we can go on.

However, false guilt is not a true indicator and can be very deceptive. If the red light on your car malfunctioned and came on, even though there was nothing actually wrong, you may be alarmed and move into unnecessary action.

False guilt is the lack in confidence in your food decision-making process. If you are a master at peace with food, you shouldn't experience false guilt. Beginners may struggle with false guilt initially but can learn to deal with it appropriately over time. Take a look at the following examples of true guilt and false guilt.

The following are examples of true guilt:
- At Thanksgiving you stuffed yourself with foods you enjoy, even though they no longer tasted good after the first serving.
- Even though you weren't hungry and didn't desire a particular food, you binged anyway.
- You felt sad, bored, or depressed, so you overate to deaden the pain.

The following are examples of false guilt:
- You feel pressure to exercise traditionally, so you sign up for an exercise class because all your friends do, but you really don't want to.
- You feel bad for eating a cheeseburger and fries (which you had planned for) because everyone else ordered salad.

- During the holidays you consumed more than you normally would. You are upset with yourself, even though you did the right thing by eating only what you desired, and you stopped when food no longer tasted good and/or before you were stuffed.

Learn to differentiate between true guilt and false guilt and feel confident in your decisions. By taking the appropriate steps to deal with that guilt, you can move on.

Healthy Foods Are No Longer a Big Deal

One thing you won't find in peace with food is a rule that says you have to eat only *healthy* foods and eliminate all *unhealthy* foods. That's because food is not the problem, but rather your relationship or bad habits with food. Besides, diets have eliminated what they considered unhealthy foods from the get-go, and with a less than one percent success rate of maintaining the weight loss, we can throw that rule out the window.

> If you abuse food, it will abuse you.

Maybe you are about to come unglued reading the above paragraph, insisting that food is the reason for your high cholesterol, high blood pressure, heart disease, and extra pounds. Your mindless eating or other bad habits are the reason for your poor health, yet the sweets, fried foods, and unhealthy food in general get the bum rap. If these foods were to blame, then everyone who eats these unhealthy foods should have the same results as yours. Let's face it, there are many people who eat these same foods and don't suffer from all the health conditions that ail overweight people.

Maybe you chalk it up to genetics. Those foods just affect you differently, you say. Well, that may be partially true, but it still comes back to the way you handle food. If you abuse food, it will abuse you.

So, if food is not the problem, are we suggesting you can eat all the unhealthy food you want? Are you off the hook for eating healthy foods? We will always encourage healthy eating, but we do realize the idea of eating only veggies, fruit, chicken, and fish doesn't always sound appealing.

Not long after embarking on our journey we found, by freeing ourselves from self-imposed food restrictions, the idea of eating healthy food wasn't so dreadful. We began eating healthier more often, not because we had to but because we wanted to, and we knew unhealthy foods weren't altogether off-limits. It became our choice, not some rule we were resentfully following. You may be surprised to find eating healthier foods could become a non-issue when you stop depriving yourself of foods you love.

Now, this doesn't mean you'll crave only healthy foods and despise unhealthy foods, however, when you allow yourself to eat the foods you love from time to time, eating foods that are more nutritionally sound won't be a big deal.

Making Healthy Choices

If you've ever bought a magazine showcasing a celebrity and their new slender body, it is usually due to a diet they recently went on. Inevitably they give a snapshot of how they eat and it always looks the same:

Breakfast: Egg white omelet with vegetables
Snack: 1 tablespoon of almond butter with celery sticks
Lunch: Chicken breast, salad, and fruit
Snack: Handful of nuts with yogurt
Dinner: Fish or some kind of lean meat and vegetables

No doubt this is a healthy way to eat, and we're not criticizing this meal plan if it brings peace and keeps you from feeling deprived. However, eating like that daily doesn't bring us peace. That plan would not keep us in the game.

You might be surprised to find that we are not going to tell you what you can and cannot eat. There are no food lists, no off-limit meals, and no rules dictating when you must eat. Sounds too good to be true, right? Well, it is too good. But it is true.

Neither of us are what you would call a health nut. We love sweets, but we understand the importance of nutritional foods and eating healthy. We have made changes, little by little, to have a healthier life-style. Here are some ways we have done that:

On non-eventful/ordinary days that don't include a celebration or special meal:
Lara: We may eat steak or grilled BBQ-chicken with steamed veggies or a salad. If we don't have any veggies on hand, we will throw together some fruit. We do eat potatoes, but not every day.

Robynn: We may have salad, pasta, and meat of some kind.

Around the house:
Lara: You will find fresh fruit in the fridge or on the counter. Bananas or grapes are a favorite during the colder months, and during the summer, strawberries are a must. I have grown to like hummus and almonds, and the kids will often eat them if I have them out. I also keep trail mix in the freezer along with a measured scoop to help with portion control.

Robynn: We have a basket of fruit on our counter to make it easily available for us to grab when we have the munchies.

When nothing sounds good, but we are hungry, we go for the healthier option, which may include:
Lara: Bananas (sometimes with peanut butter), carrots with ranch dressing, cheese or turkey slices, or homemade energy bites.

Robynn: Fruit of some kind. I don't want to spend a lot of calories on snacks. I want to save them for my meals. In Weight Watchers®, fruits and veggies don't have any "points" so I eat up on those.

Being farm girls, we love fresh fruits and veggies from the garden. During the summer months:
Lara: We use these fresh foods by eating a lot of chicken wraps, stuffed with tomatoes and lettuce. We also eat a lot of salads and try to be creative with different variations so we don't get burned-out. Putting strawberries in our salad is a nice treat.

Robynn: Many times during the harvest season our meal may consist of all tomatoes, cucumbers, or fruit smoothies.

We both live in small towns, so we are limited in restaurant selections. When we plan to eat out with our family:
Lara and Robynn: Try to eat lightly for the other meals of the day. If we eat out for lunch and aren't hungry for dinner, we may eliminate that meal for the evening. We eat similarly on holidays such as Thanksgiving, Christmas, and Easter.

Lara: We order carryout Chinese food sometimes. We always get one order of General Tso's Chicken with rice and then steam our own veggies at home. By adding our own vegetables, we bulk up each serving, which adds extra nutrition and stretches one order to feed our entire family.

Robynn: I may have a protein shake or Greek yogurt for breakfast.

What about water?
Lara: I should probably drink more water than I do. If I remember to fill my thirty-two-ounce mug each morning, I am more likely to drink more throughout the day. To help with my intake, I try to take a drink of water between bites at mealtime. It not only cleanses my palate and increases my water intake for the day, but it helps me get fuller faster during mealtime.

Robynn: I make water more enticing by reusing the large Styrofoam cup and straw from Sonic, a fast-food restaurant. It's funny how my kids always want to drink out of my cup.

Both of our families enjoy fruit smoothies during the hot summer. Our favorite smoothie combos include:
Lara: A blend of fresh bananas, frozen strawberries, vanilla yogurt, and milk.

Robynn: Bananas, fresh fruit, frozen fruit for thickening, and milk.

Other ways we eat healthy:
Lara:
- When we go places, I know someone in my family is going to get hungry before we make it home. I stash items in my purse such as bananas, granola bars, and water (good thing big purses are in style!) This satisfies our hunger and keeps us from being tempted by the drive-through route or grab unhealthy food at a convenience store.
- We don't always crave the healthier choice when we get hungry throughout the day, so we try to include things

that make it more enticing. A few candy sprinkles in the yogurt for the kids, or lightly drizzle chocolate syrup over peanut butter and a banana always does the trick in our house.

Robynn:

- When I go grocery shopping, I let my kids pick out a piece of fruit and a bottle of water. They feel like they are getting a treat, and it's not candy from the checkout aisle.
- I like the Weight Watchers® plan as it gives me boundaries of twenty-six points, yet gives me freedom by not telling me what to eat and when. And best of all, I'm not deprived of the foods I love.
- I like chocolate protein shakes for breakfast because they pack a big punch of protein, but are only five Weight Watchers® points.
- I put out veggies while I cook so we will snack on them rather than the food we are cooking.
- I am constantly looking for tasty recipes that include things we're not all that fond of such as broccoli and cauliflower. It is amazing what a little olive oil, breadcrumbs, and spices will do to veggies that otherwise taste bland to the palate.

Lara and Robynn:

- When it comes to your health, it is up to you and your physician to determine which route will be best for you. Maybe counting calories will work best or utilizing the plan many dietitians use: divide your plate into fourths and place one serving of protein (the size of a small fist), carbohydrates, fruit, and vegetables on each quadrant.

- Find ways to increase the consumption of healthy foods and water. One way is to make it easily accessible. When our kids see us eat these foods, they want some as well. If you or your kids get food cravings between the time they get home from school and dinner, set out fruit slices and carrots. Remember, if unhealthy foods are out of sight, they will more likely be out of mind.

We hope our answers will help you come up with your own tailor-made lifestyle to encourage healthy eating. By no means do we eat this way every day, and we certainly don't stick to only these ideas. Keep in mind, these are ways we try to fit healthy foods into our individual lifestyles. What you feel is attainable will be up to you.

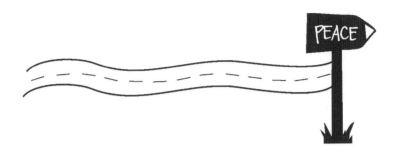

N. Roadside Fruit Stand

Healthy Eating—What are you already doing that promotes healthy eating?

- _____
- _____
- _____
- _____
- _____
- _____
- _____

What is one way you can include a new healthy selection in your day?

- _____
- _____
- _____
- _____
- _____
- _____
- _____

What are you already doing that promotes healthy eating?
Lara: I make homemade energy bites on Sunday evenings and freeze them so they are easily accessible for breakfast each morning. This keeps me from being tempted to eat an unhealthier option such as Pop-Tart or sugary

cereal. We also make a point to eat some type of fruit or vegetable with every meal.

Robynn: Starting out the day with a healthy meal, drinking water, and having fruits and veggies easily accessible.

What is one way you can include a new healthy selection in your day?
Lara: By planning ahead what I am going to eat for lunch. Since I stay at home with the kids, it is easy for me to grab food that is not always a healthy option, because it is easier to prepare versus a salad. Since I take the time to make energy bites on Sunday evenings for the upcoming week of breakfasts, maybe I should consider preparing healthy lunch options as well.

Robynn: I struggle with eating a variety of vegetables. Each year my goal is to eat more vegetables than I did the year before.

Chapter 8 Take-Home Messages

✓Eating what you love, using wisdom and moderation, can actually help you lose the extra weight.

✓Eat whatever you want, as long as it brings you peace.

✓Peace with food gives you permission to have a psychological release.

✓It's simple math: if you substitute your binging by allowing yourself to have what you really want and what gives peace, it will have a positive impact on your scale.

✓Identify the reasons you eat out of bounds and then make efforts to correct those bad habits by developing new and better habits.

✓Hitting the bullseye of peace with food will take a lot of target practice, but over time it will result in precision!

✓True guilt shines a light on a problem so you can fix it and move on. False guilt is due to the expectations of yourself or others and only condemns you.

✓Peace with food isn't about eating only healthy foods. It's about learning to eat foods in their appropriate portions.

✓Create your own plan for eating healthy and nutritional foods.

CHAPTER

9

Food (B)

Enjoying Comfort Food

Robynn

There she was in all her glory and grace. Ms. Trisha Yearwood cooking away on the Food Network. It was the first time I'd seen her cooking show, and I was transfixed. Her comfort and ease in front of the camera reeled me in. It was as if I were right there, sitting on the other side of her island while she shared her dad's famous Brunswick stew recipe.

As she taught her nephews the recipe for their grandfather's famous stew, the three of them talked about the good memories they had of this beloved man. This was not just another recipe. It was a dish jam-packed with fond memories, deliciousness, and comfort. Comfort southern style.

And then Trisha unpacked the powerful truth behind the definition of comfort food: "The reason it's called comfort food is because it not only nourishes the body, but it comforts the soul."

Ding. Ding. Ding. Ding. Bingo!

Trisha nailed it on the head. *Comfort Food* comforts the soul.

This is one reason diets fail. They ignore this very basic premise—that eating is not just an activity that nourishes the body; it also nourishes the soul. When you are forced to eat food you don't like and are prohibited from eating food you enjoy, an emotional/psychological void is created. Eventually that void will be filled, and usually that results in an uncontrollable binge.

Comfort food is a good thing. A really, really, good thing. When used properly (to fuel the body while comforting the soul) and within the appropriate boundaries, comfort food can be, well, comforting.

Comfort food can also be abused, especially when people try to use food to comfort themselves when food is not the answer. That does not mean comfort food is bad.

Sometimes the comforting factor behind comfort food is not necessarily the food, but rather the combination of factors such as the food, people, and the event. When you take away any one of those factors, the comfort is gone.

Lara and I absolutely love everything about Thanksgiving, including our favorite dishes. However, if we made those same dishes in June and served them to our families, they wouldn't have the same meaning. In fact, we might not even classify them as comfort food at that time because these foods are all about enjoying them on this special holiday—time with our extended families, football on the television interspersed with Christmas commercials, and cool weather blustering outside.

Think about comfort food in your life. Maybe you have never defined it as such, but you have events in your life when you gather with family or friends and eat. Your families enjoy Christmas together with a feast fit for a king, or there are settings where you only eat certain foods and only in that setting, such as on holidays or special occasions or in certain locations. If the setting is pleasant, no doubt you probably associate good feelings with these foods.

Think back to when you were a child. You probably have memories of eating a certain food with certain people in certain settings. Years may pass without your eating that food, but the instant you do, those memories are immediately recalled. That is the power of comfort food.

We recognize the importance of comfort food and are going to spend this chapter sharing the tools we use to enjoy food in a way that gives peace. The food that nourishes your body, comforts your soul, and gives you great happiness as you celebrate the special moments of your life with those you love.

And speaking of comfort food, let's take a break at our next rest stop!

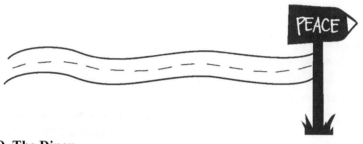

O. The Diner
Comfort Food—What is your comfort food?

- _____
- _____
- _____
- _____
- _____
- _____
- _____

Lara: My husband's chocolate chip cookies right out of the oven, Chinese take-out, appetizers like chips and dip, coffee, stuffing at Thanksgiving, and my Grandma's homemade chicken and noodles.

Robynn: The Thanksgiving meal. Fried chicken, mashed potatoes with gravy, and corn. Sweet stuff like pecan pie, pumpkin pie, apple dumplings, cheesecake, Peanut Butter and Chocolate Girl Scout Cookies, Kid's Meal Bacon Cheeseburger and French Fries with Lemonade from Dairy Queen, and the German food I grew up on.

Don't Waste Your Calories

Lara

I can think of countless times I have eaten things placed in front of me, not because I loved how it tasted, but because it was easily available. So often our minds are on autopilot and we don't even think about what we are putting into our mouths. We just eat because it is convenient and it gives some type of temporary satisfaction whether we actually love the food or not.

Our tool, *Don't Waste Your Calories*, has probably been the area where I get my biggest payoff. Once I realized I was eating hundreds of calories on foods and drinks I was mindlessly consuming, it helped me shed some extra weight and made me appreciate the foods I did choose to spend my calories on. I have even gone so far as to spit food out if I taste it and don't love it. I figure if it didn't satisfy my taste buds once it hit my tongue, there was no point in consuming the extra calories. Obviously in a group setting, it would be rude to spit something out

> **The Exception**
>
> Fruits and vegetables are the exception to not wasting your calories, because they pack a punch nutritionally and are relatively low in calories. Fish, lean proteins, nuts, and legumes also fall in this category. These foods make the best use of your calories while also fueling the body.

because you don't like it. You may need to make exceptions when you are around other people. But don't feel bad about doing it in situations that are appropriate.

"I'll just eat ice cream and chips every day since that is all I really enjoy," you say. Well, not so fast. We encourage healthy eating, so it is important not to use the don't-waste-your-calories concept as an excuse to eat poorly. If you don't like eating vegetables or drinking water, we are not saying you should eliminate those things from your life. What we are saying is you should double check that everything you put in your mouth is worth consuming. A vegetable or fruit is worth eating because you know it has nutritional benefits, but grabbing a couple of cold French fries as you get up from the dinner table is often wasted calories. You are probably only eating them because they are still *there*. The food was available to you, so you ate it, whether it served a purpose or not. Instead, you could have saved those meaningless calories and used them on something you really cherished.

Let's say you go to work and sit down to eat your favorite breakfast food: a chocolate protein bar. Before you can take your awaited first bite, you get called to a staff meeting. When you arrive in the conference room, you see bagels and fruit. You go over and have a bagel because it is available. Even though you don't love bagels, they are free and can be yours in a matter of seconds. "I *am* hungry," you say to yourself, but you never think twice about going for the fruit because carbs are your kryptonite.

As an alternative to eating the bagel, you could have eaten several slices of fruit to tide you over (which we don't consider wasted calories), and then used your calories on the food you enjoy most. Instead, you probably mindlessly ate a free bagel *and* fruit, both of which you didn't love, and then ended up eating the protein bar when you returned to your desk, because that is what you were craving all along. Look how many calories could have been saved.

Not wasting your calories also applies to food you love but don't desire at the time. Remember your favorite chocolate cake that you ate on your anniversary. You savored every bite the night of the party, but now it is hanging around for a second day and a third day...and you keep eating it even though you no longer desire it. Put an end to the craziness!

Don't waste any more calories by mindlessly eating. Take a second to evaluate what you put in your mouth and make every calorie count.

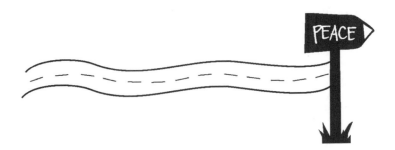

P. Waste Management

Eliminating foods that are a waste of calories—What foods could you eliminate that are a waste of calories?

- _____
- _____
- _____
- _____
- _____
- _____
- _____

Lara:
- The crust on a pizza.
- Eating what is left on my kid's plate.
- Taking more than one taste test while cooking dinner.
- Eating leftovers from dinner as I put food away.
- Eating food that is burnt or has a bad aftertaste. (Dinner I ruined but still eat because of the time I spent cooking it.)

Robynn:
- Having an adult burger or chicken strip meal when a kid's meal would have satisfied me instead.

- Whipped cream. Because I don't feel the need to have it, I leave it off.
- Caloric drinks, with the exception of special events.
- Seconds—unless it is a once a year meal, such as Thanksgiving.

Like-It and Love-It Foods

Lara

Close your eyes. Picture a special occasion when you are gathering with your closest friends and family for a feast. You knock on the front door, walk through the foyer, and spot the table. It is beautifully set with mouthwatering dishes of your favorite foods. Foods that you *love*. As you step closer to get a better look, your eyes skim the array of your most desired indulgences. So what are they exactly? Could you list all of your favorite foods that were on that table?

Figuring out what foods you really *love* versus only *like* will be helpful so you don't end up wasting your calories on foods that won't get the appreciation they deserve. Peace with food allows you to eat what you want, as long as it gives you peace, and you'll find the foods that fall in this category are either your absolute favorites or are healthy and nutritious for your body. Foods that give you peace usually aren't just mediocre to the taste buds and/or to your overall health (at least they aren't for us!).

If we laid twenty candy bars in front of you and asked you to record your favorite, it might be too hard to choose just one. It is difficult to narrow it down to one because they all look so good! As a result, you may be tempted to write down (and eat) several of them. Differentiating between foods we like and love can be hard for some people because we think we love them all. But at the heart of our desires, we really only love certain dishes. And when we take the time to discover these love-it dishes, we can train our mind to block out the cravings for all the other like-it items on our list.

Another thing to consider is the temperature of the food you are eating or the environment in which you are eating. For example, I love pizza when it is hot, but if it is room temperature, I only like it. When it is Christmastime, I love hot chocolate, but any other time of year, I only like it. I have learned that I don't even bother eating pizza unless it is warmed up to the temperature I prefer, and I only keep hot chocolate on hand during the month of December. Don't limit yourself only to the foods themselves. Consider all angles before you decide how you truly feel about them.

And instead of walking to your pantry or fridge to try to figure out what sounds good, really think about past experiences and foods that you truly enjoyed and loved. We usually get different results when we are presented with too many options, so if certain favorite foods don't come to mind initially, you may want to think twice about eating them. If you are anything like us, you are probably just eating some foods because it is "there" and easily available, not because you actually love them.

Mr. Right vs. Mr. Right-Now

When it comes to finding the right guy, you may have heard the phrase *Mr. Right vs. Mr. Right-Now* (the same applies to men and Mrs. Right). Mr. Right refers to marrying a man truly right for you, whereas Mr. Right-Now describes a man who is the best pick at that time due to accessibility. In other words, he is right there.

Food presents a similar scenario. We have discovered two kinds of desires involved in eating: a Mr. Right desire and a Mr. Right-Now desire. Here is the following description of each:

Mr. Right:
- It is a craving that doesn't go away.
- It exists even if you are not around food.
- Walking away from the temptation leaves you feeling deprived.
- Giving yourself permission to enjoy food you truly desire in a controlled manner brings satisfaction and curbs the desire.

Mr. Right-Now
- It is short-lived.
- It is temporary and exists because you are around food or because food is easily accessible and has become a

temptation. The moment you get away from the food, the desire vanishes.
* Walking away from the temptation leaves you feeling victorious rather than deprived.

Mr. Right-Now is a short-term desire, so one strategy to avoid this bad eating habit is to get away from the food that is tempting you. If you are like many people, avoiding easily accessible food is a challenge. You can sometimes use Mr. Right-Now to your advantage by surrounding yourself with healthy and nutritious food. Chances are, if it is available, you'll be more likely to eat it, and this can help you achieve a well-balanced diet if you have difficulty eating enough fruits and vegetables. In this case, Mr. Right-Now can actually be a good thing.

Satisfy a legitimate need by having a plan. Plans need to have allowances for the food you desire. If you desire a candy bar, prepare to take a 30-minute brisk walk in addition to your daily exercise. If you desire sitting down to enjoy your family's yearly Christmas feast, you may decide to eat light for the other meals that day and/or exercise ahead of time.

Next time you have a desire to eat something that's not part of your plan for that day, ask yourself if you are facing a Mr. Right-Now desire or a legitimate Mr. Right desire. Once you have identified what type of desire you are facing, you can take the necessary steps to arrive at a place of freedom and peace.

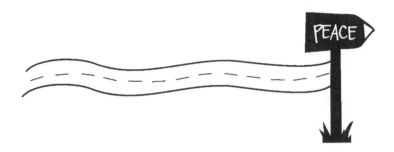

Q. Wedding Chapel

Food Preferences—What is your *Mr. Right* when it comes to food?
(Your favorite foods.)

- _____
- _____
- _____
- _____
- _____
- _____
- _____

What is your *Mr. Right-Now* when it comes to food? (Foods you
eat because they are easily accessible.)

- _____
- _____
- _____
- _____
- _____
- _____
- _____

What is your *Mr. Right* when it comes to food? (Your favorite
foods.)

Lara: My favorite healthy foods consist of
hummus with almonds, frozen trail mix, and
sweet peppers with ranch dressing. For
occasional special treats I like chocolate,

anything sweet, salty things, a good steak or burger, carbs, or take-out food.

Robynn: My favorite healthy foods are fresh tomatoes from the garden, fresh strawberries, peaches, mangos, and watermelon. For main dishes, I like turkey burgers, chicken fajitas, and fish tacos. For a light meal, I like California Rolls and Spring Rolls, and my husband's green leaf salads with homemade dressing. For occasional special treats, I prefer sweet stuff like cookie dough, pies, and pastries.

What is your *Mr. Right-Now* when it comes to food? (Foods you eat because they are easily accessible.)
Lara: Again, usually leftovers that my kids don't eat. Ack!

Robynn: Snack food such as pretzels, crackers, and second helpings.

Bite #1 vs. Bite #21

Lara
A glass full of chocolate milk. Warm maple syrup. Buttery homemade pancakes. These are three things that describe the flavors I anticipated for weeks. My son's birthday had finally arrived, and we were going to celebrate it at our favorite breakfast joint. That's right, my taste buds were so enthralled that I began salivating just thinking about it as we pulled out of our driveway and headed into town.

The moment came and I reached for my fork…

- Bite #1: AWESOME.
- Bite #2: YUM…need I say more?
- Bite #4: Still, *really* good.
- Bite #10: Wow, I can't believe I've eaten only one

fourth of this enormous short stack! Need to add more syrup.

- Bite #15: *Sigh.* Perhaps I am getting full. But wait. I dreamed about this meal for days. I owe this to myself to keep eating.
- Bite #21: Why…why did I do this to myself? I am so stuffed that all I want to do is go home and go to bed.

Now take a look at that series of bites again. That first bite—wow—kind of hard to beat! Even at bite #4, it still tasted *really* good. But by bite #10, I wasn't even thinking about how good it tasted. In fact, I was already in the mindset of persevering to finish it.

There is a great lie that people who struggle with food tend to believe: If one serving is good, then two, three, or more is even better.

Although this sounds logical, it simply is not true. Our bodies were designed in the exact opposite way. Food tastes best when we are hungry. The satisfaction we get from food doesn't increase as we get full, but diminishes with every bite.

You may have heard of the principle in economics called *The Law of Diminishing Returns*. In a nutshell, increasing production while everything else remains constant eventually decreases returns. In this case, the production is the food you eat, and the return is the satisfaction you receive from it. Initially the satisfaction may be great, but the more you eat, the less satisfaction you receive.

At first this concept was foreign to us, but we now understand the insidious lie that if one serving is great then two must be better.

As kids we were taught always to clean our plates. This meant forcing ourselves to finish even though it didn't bring peace or satisfaction. So if bite #21 doesn't taste as good as bite #1, don't feel obligated to finish your meal. Yes, wasting food is not ideal, but managing your weight is more important. Plus, the more you learn at which bite the food loses its appeal, you'll learn to adjust your portion sizes accordingly.

This is often a factor when you go out to eat. You can order what you like, knowing you don't have to polish off the entire plate (unless you planned for it). Rather, you can split your meal with a friend, take part of it home, or leave a portion of it on the plate. Dining out doesn't have to be a daunting task, especially when you have a plan.

If you want peace with food, you will have to use the law of diminishing returns to your advantage. It takes time, patience, and practice. You won't do this perfectly when you begin. Many times it will feel like you take one step forward and three backwards. Although frustrating, it is a normal part of the process. We spent a lot of time developing this skill. We fell down often, but got up each time, refusing to quit. So, don't be discouraged if you don't do it perfectly. With every aim at the target, you are getting closer. So keep aiming.

Have Closure with Food

Do not plan for ventures before finishing what's at hand.
~Euripides

Lara

I think of the word *Closure* as saying, "Goodbye" to something for the last time. In relationships, once you have closure, you can move on. The same applies to food.

Closure might be finishing off your favorite bag of potato chips or eating the last bite of apple pie. From your first bite to your last, your body goes through a process that prepares itself for the final bite. If you can train your mind into experiencing closure in all things you eat, you will consume fewer calories, which results in faster weight loss.

Let's say a person loves brownies. In this case, a fresh pan hot from the oven may be a dangerous temptation. After the first bite of this decadent treat, the pull may be too great to stop with the first piece. After all, there is nothing more enticing than an unfinished pan of brownies! By training your mind to experience closure, you can walk away in peace, even in difficult situations such as this. Instead of staring at an unfinished pan of brownies, cut an acceptable-sized piece and hide the rest away in the cabinet or back in the oven. Once the brownie is gone, your eyes see an empty plate, and your mind can move on.

We know this can be easier said than done, and it may require a little extra discipline to have a successful closure experience with food. When I get lazy and think I have enough control, I still end up eating more than I planned because it is too hard to walk away from a half-eaten bag of chips. In extreme cases I may make a batch of cookies, put a few on a plate, and throw the rest away. From countless experiences, if I keep them around, I won't feel closure until they are gone.

Closure can be an excellent tool for eating in moderation. It can provide a great sense of satisfaction, right down to the last bite. Consider using it the next time you grab something to eat.

Recognize When You Need a Break

Lara

While working on this book, I became pregnant with our third child. When I was twenty-four weeks pregnant, my doctor recommended I watch my sugar intake because I barely passed my glucose screening. He put me on a low-carb diet for the final fourteen weeks of my pregnancy, so you can imagine my desire to overindulge in sweets and breads. I didn't even have to ask. The morning after we had our son, my husband handed me two apple fritters and a container of chocolate milk. I was in heaven!

Once I returned home, I told Robynn I planned to give myself a break regarding food. I assumed I would eat whatever I wanted for a week and easily bounce back into eating healthy and normal. In anticipation of this free week, I even froze some of my favorite Christmas candy in December, knowing a month later I could finally eat it.

My "vacation" lasted days, then weeks, and before I knew it, two months had passed. I still felt like I was making up for lost time, eating whatever I wanted, as much as I wanted, whenever I wanted. The last thing on my mind was getting back on track with food. Recovering from having a baby and being incredibly sleep-deprived, I just wasn't *there*.

Occasionally it takes time to get the ball rolling in the right direction. And then it happened. I finally experienced the straw that broke the camel's back: chocolate-covered popcorn. That delicacy had been calling my name since Christmas, and it was on my list of things to make once the baby arrived. After picking my son up from preschool, the craving instantly hit me. On a whim, I raced to the grocery store to purchase all the ingredients.

At home, I threw everything together and began eating before the dessert was even complete. I had made an entire batch and, before I knew it, had eaten over half of it!

Sadly, being stuffed didn't stop me from eating more, and I could see I was headed down a disastrous road. I left the room and had a stern talk with myself. I knew all the benefits of our concept, but it didn't stop me from shoving more chocolate almond bark into my mouth. Eating it wasn't giving me peace, yet I did it anyway.

I decided enough was enough. I grabbed the bowl, threw it in the trash, slammed the lid, and said, "I'm done!" Instantly I felt better. That defining moment finally got me back on track with eating after months of consuming junk food. It was as if slamming the lid on the trash can showed the food who was boss.

Next time you feel like you're drowning in defeat, consider doing something radical enough to get your focus back in the right direction. It is amazing how taking a hammer to the scale or ripping the tags out of your jeans will give you a fresh start.

Create Situations You Can Control

Robynn

All my life, I had certain foods that seemed to dominate me. Anytime they were available, they had the upper hand. They always won the fight.

One day after binging on a rich dessert, date balls, I'd had enough. I said aloud, "You will not defeat me! I will defeat you!"

From that moment on, I was on a mission. I would find a way to eat date balls and not binge. As I began to construct my plan, I realized I lacked self-control. These rich and gooey treats were so delicious. Controlling myself while mixing a skillet full of this yummy concoction on the stovetop was nearly impossible.

So, the question came to mind: What if I cut the recipe down five times to fit within the amount of calories I chose to spend? I would only be making the amount of date balls I had preplanned to eat.

The result: it worked like a charm. I found my answer to a problem that had plagued me for decades. In this simple experiment, I learned how to eat whatever food I desire by taking authority over the food instead of letting it take authority over me. When I did, I realized the foods that once controlled me had been disarmed. It allowed me to eat them with peace and walk away without guilt. That, my friends, is an inbounds psychological release.

Now it's your turn. Take the food that trips you up and cut the recipe or portions down to the appropriate size. Maybe that means only eating a third of a cheeseburger or a half piece of cheesecake. Whatever it is, take control of the situation by having a plan that stays within your boundaries. When you do, you will be creating experiences that work in your favor, disarming the foods that control you.

Get Rid of Temptation

Lara

Have you ever tried to break a bad habit, but the habit is always staring you down? I remember having this issue with a red velvet cake. Although I knew a tremendous number of calories are in every slice and how sluggish it made me feel after I ate it, I still wanted more.

My solution was to throw the cake away. I enjoyed two generous slices over the weekend, but I won't feel guilty for throwing something away that is only going to make me feel worse. Back in the day, I would have never thought to do such a thing. Knowing there are starving people in the world or that I was throwing money away would have kept me from tossing that cake. However, keeping unnecessary snacks and junk food around the house would just be contributing to another big problem in this country, weight management.

Sometimes we have to take extreme measures to avoid being stared down by our temptations. In the end, we need to do whatever it takes to set ourselves up to succeed, even if it means tossing out our favorite desserts after we've had our fill. Quit worrying about food going to waste and learn to be okay with throwing out food that is going to *your* waist. *Wink.*

Restaurants and Travel

Both of our families travel a few times a year, so when we do, we want to enjoy the time spent together. During our travels, we try not to worry about what we eat; however, we do try to eat smart when we can. We eat small at breakfast (breakfast bar, cereal, granola, or fruit) and then have one large meal that day. If the big meal is at lunch, we eat light for supper and vice versa. We don't give ourselves a license to eat excessively. We try to eat healthy when possible, but if there's something we want to eat, we eat it. No one wants to visit new places and not be able to enjoy their authentic dishes!

When Robynn is traveling by car, she likes to get an egg and cheese biscuit from McDonald's® for breakfast. It brings back memories of traveling home to South Dakota from Kansas during the summer with her cousin Rachelle. She continues this tradition—maybe two or three times a year—because it meets a psychological need for her.

As a child, Lara grew up going on family vacations every summer. Their trips usually involved visiting a national park. Prior to leaving, her family would pack food for their entire trip. They would eat breakfast consisting of cereal, toast, or fruit in the hotel room. For lunch they would typically stop and have a picnic with a sandwich, chips, and candy bar. Since breakfast and lunch were fairly small meals, dinner would usually be the biggest meal of the day at a restaurant.

Now that Lara has a family of her own, they continue the tradition of packing meals in advance. Since they travel with picnic food, she makes a point *not* to stow it in the front seat of the car. If she does allow snack food up front, she only takes a small portion and leaves the rest in the trunk. That way, the temptation is more of an inconvenience to get to.

Lara's husband, Doug, has a job that requires a lot of road time. Many days he does not take his lunch. If he wants fast food, he tries to watch his portion size or eats at Subway. With smaller portion sizes, he can get closure by eating the entire meal without feeling guilty. If he goes out for lunch, he usually eats light for the remainder of the day.

Robynn's husband, Scott, also travels some. Instead of eating fast food, he packs a protein bar, shake, or sandwich from home to eat on the road.

Speaking of traveling, stopping to eat at a restaurant can be a dieter's downfall. Thankfully, we are not dieters, so restaurants are no longer a landmine. Still, we have strategies to help keep us on track. Here are some of those strategies:

- We plan ahead and know what we're going to eat. Usually we'll eat smaller meals the rest of the day, so we can enjoy the dining out experience.
- We try to eat a small snack prior to eating out. We've learned if we allow ourselves to get too hungry, we overeat at the restaurant and don't make good choices.
- To work our principle of closure to our advantage, we order kid's meals whenever possible or share a meal with someone. Instead of ordering the large value-size meal, we pick the smallest option available. This allows us to enjoy the food we desire but doesn't waste our calories.
- Get a to-go box. Lara and her family don't mind leftovers. If this is you, remember: your first bite of food will always taste the best, so when the newness has worn off and/or you become full, ask the server for a to-go box. It may not be as fresh tomorrow, but to some degree, you will get to experience that first bite again. You won't waste your calories and can stretch your savored meal for another day.
- If going to a chain restaurant, we may look up the nutritional information and decide what to order ahead of time.
- If we are indifferent about what sounds good, we opt for the healthier choice, such as loading up on veggies as a substitute for potatoes.

- Occasionally, if there is something we really want, we allow ourselves to indulge and enjoy, within boundaries, of course.

Traveling and restaurants do not need to be failure traps. When eating out, you can eliminate temptation by being prepared. Trying to come up with a plan as you gaze at a menu is not a wise strategy. Have a plan before you even step foot in the restaurant or hit the road, and you'll be more likely to make better decisions.

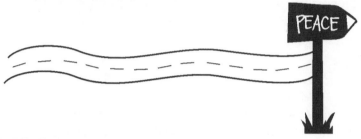

R. The Restaurant

Eating-Out Strategy—What are some strategies you can use to successfully eat in peace while you are eating out or traveling?

- _____
- _____
- _____
- _____
- _____
- _____
- _____

Lara: Anything goes, but I do try to eat a meal that has fruits and vegetables or is high in fiber. Overall, enjoy the trip but don't waste calories on food or drinks you don't love. For long road trips, leave the snacks in the trunk and only grab enough to satisfy and give closure.

Lara and Robynn: We plan ahead and eat smaller portions for the other meals of the day and eat an occasional snack to avoid entering the restaurant on an empty stomach (which usually causes us to overeat because we are famished). Enjoy the dining experience and eat what we want, maybe just not the entire portion. We don't waste our calories on food that doesn't meet our expectations. If one of the side dishes doesn't taste as good as we'd hoped, we don't feel obligated to eat it.

Embrace Special Occasions

"It's the most wonderful time of the year…" However, if you're on a diet, your version may go more like this: "It's the most tormenting time of the year…"

As much as we love cake at a wedding or nachos while watching the Super Bowl, it can be detrimental if we don't have a plan. In addition to these special occasions, there will also be unexpected situations that arise. Think of the friend who pops in and surprises you with your favorite milkshake or the impromptu party at work. What do you do then?

At one time, before our journey, our strategy was to either refrain from the food at these special times or indulge in the food and be tortured with guilt because it was against our current diet.

We realized that passing up the opportunity to eat during these out-of-the-ordinary events always left us feeling deprived. And you know what deprivation will do…it comes back to haunt you. Within days we would regret not eating the food we craved at the occasion, so we would try replacing it by eating whatever we could scrounge up at home. This never worked because the moment had already passed. Had we allowed ourselves to eat the special dessert Grandma makes exclusively for baby showers or the ice cream that's only available in grocery stores at Christmastime, we could have enjoyed it, filled a need, and moved on. Instead, we not only missed out but ended up consuming way more calories days later, trying to make up for lost time and food! It's madness, we tell you. Madness!

The holidays and special occasions are a fun time to gather with friends and family. Since holidays can be tricky, we have included how we handle them. Let's take a look at what may (or may not) work for you:

- We plan ahead. When we know there will be a big meal, whether it is a holiday or not, we try to eat lightly for the other two meals.
- We make a conscious effort to avoid mindless eating by not grazing on food that is *Mr. Right-Now* and only eat food that is *Mr. Right*. To help with this we:
  - o Try to keep something to drink in one hand as we focus on family and conversation.
  - o Remove ourselves from the kitchen or areas that have food sitting out, unless it is mealtime.
- Give ourselves the sweets or holiday foods we desire. We do it with a plan, such as stopping when we are full or enjoying mini-slices of our favorite desserts.

As for those unexpected experiences, just go with them. Those are special moments you'll never get back, so allow yourself to indulge during those occasions as well. That doesn't mean overindulge and give yourself a license to pork out and lose control. Instead, treat it like a psychological release and eat in ways that give peace.

Jot down some ideas you could implement at this next rest stop.

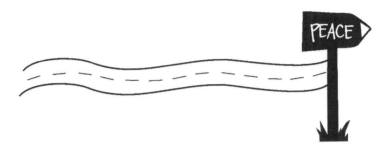

S. The Christmas Store
Holiday Strategy—How can you eat during the holidays in a way that will bring your soul comfort, but also peace?

- _____
- _____
- _____
- _____
- _____
- _____
- _____

Lara and Robynn: We try to eat lightly leading up to the holidays. When the holidays arrive, we give ourselves permission to enjoy the meals and get back to our regular eating when they are over. We eat smart by skimping during those times when our family is not having a feast. However, when there is food we love, we eat what we want and stop when food doesn't taste good to us anymore.

Adjust When Plans Change

Lara

When I became pregnant while working on this book, I understood the importance of creating a lifestyle that gives peace. As I mentioned earlier, at twenty-four weeks pregnant, I took the glucose screening and barely passed. Due to the borderline results, my doctor decided I should cut back on carbs for the duration of my pregnancy just to play it safe. Not exactly something I was excited about with Halloween, Thanksgiving, and Christmas rapidly approaching.

Thankfully, I had been living at peace with food for a couple of years, so I didn't panic when realizing I was limited to a fifteen-gram carb allotment for all meals and snacks. Believe me, this did not allow much room for fun foods. However, I was determined to make my pregnancy as enjoyable as possible despite my restrictions. I had no other choice. I wasn't about to put my baby or my own health in danger.

The first thing I did was talk to my sister, who had already gone through gestational diabetes. She was extremely helpful in sharing her go-to snacks. I also spent time at the grocery store finding foods that stayed within my diet, but also sounded tasty. When I went home, I sampled the different items and kept only what I enjoyed. Eating what I liked would help me stay on track, and I didn't want to waste calories on foods I had to choke down. Sure, some of the low calorie brownie snacks didn't taste as good as my favorite brownie recipe, but I was happy to find something that satisfied my sweet tooth while staying within my carb allowance.

I learned that being patient and finding what I liked was extremely beneficial to my success. Prior to this experience, I'd never been a hummus fan. After trying different flavors, I was able to find hummus I enjoyed. I also discovered I liked dipping it with almonds, which was a healthier alternative than chips! Believe it or not, I continue to eat it that way today.

Life can throw us curveballs. Sometimes we have to follow a specific eating plan because that's what the doctor ordered. This can be a major disappointment. But by living at peace with food the transition to making prescribed changes should be easier since you are learning to be adaptable and flexible. If your doctor has put you on a specific eating plan, but you really miss a few of your regular must-have foods, talk to your doctor and see if you can enjoy them occasionally.

Indulge Without Sacrificing Peace

The following is a blog post from one of our favorite bloggers, Layla Palmer of *The Lettered Cottage*. We were so tickled when we read the following post that we thought we would share. When you walk in peace with food you can have the kind of adventure she talks about. Back in our dieting days, this would have taken us over the edge. These days, we know we have the freedom to experience this kind of indulgence from time to time. We hope you enjoy it as much as we did![6]

On February 1, 2013, Layla writes:

The following texts were exchanged between me and my neighbor/BFF on January 26, at 8:52pm. My texts are dark gray, hers are light gray:

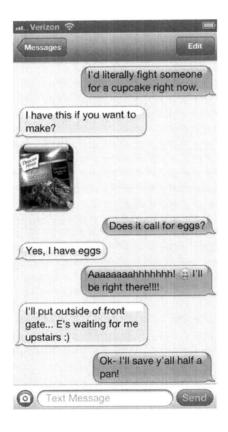

Getting a sweet tooth craving late at night when you've already got your PJ's on and don't feel like going to the store: NOT GOOD.

Having a friend who will share brownie mix and organic eggs with you before she heads upstairs to tuck in her little one: PRICELESS!

Eating so much brownie batter you're not even hungry for the actual brownies when they're done cooling: TYPICAL.

Have you made anything sweet lately? If so, leave me a link! I'm "paper pregnant" and expect to have a few more late-night sweet tooth cravings this year.

Layla

Allow Yourself to Eat Food You Love

Robynn

Before I began my peace with food journey, the holidays were accompanied by cruddy feelings of defeat and despair. If you haven't noticed by now, I love sweets, absolutely love them!

Here's the truth: Back then, cookie dough used to be one of my favorite *foods*—yes , I know some people wouldn't consider it a food, but I do. All my life, I have felt like a closet cookie dough eater. I didn't want anyone to know how much I loved this stuff because, if you are an overeater and have issues with food, at least be dignified enough to have an obsession with pizza or ice cream. But cookie dough? After all, you can justify eating a bacon double cheeseburger, fries, and a Coke when you are hungry, but justifying eating cookie dough is a stretch. The funny thing is, since embarking on my journey to peace with food, I have met numerous people who love cookie dough. It turns out I wasn't that different after all.

One of my biggest triggers leading me to overeat cookie dough was seeing a picture of sugar cookie dough rolled out on a floured pastry mat complete with cookie cutouts. This got me every time. When I saw this image, it was like Pavlov's dogs—my mouth would start watering, my eyes would get bigger, and my stomach started growling.

Perhaps I had this obsession not only because I loved the taste, but it also took me back to being a kid and making these cookies with my mom. Very often we would have Christmas music playing in the background and Christmas aromas wafting through the kitchen. As a result, sugar cookies are a comfort food for me.

During the holidays, I felt even more tormented as television commercials and magazines always included pictures of rolled out sugar cookie dough. Here I was, a grown woman fantasizing about sugar cookie dough on a well-floured countertop. I felt defeated and hopeless, and to drown out all the pain I ate even more cookie dough.

When I finally began my journey I was determined to no longer be defeated. I can now say, with a big sigh, "Mission accomplished." These days, I give myself cookie dough whenever I desire it, but only with a plan. I stay within my boundaries most of the time by sticking to my Weight Watchers® points. This results in not only satisfying a desire, but also self-control and freedom.

Incidentally, once I gave myself the thing I truly desired in moderation and under control, I found that the gravitational pull to cookie dough virtually disappeared.

This doesn't mean I don't like cookie dough anymore. I still like it, but now that I know it is available to me whenever I desire it—Christmas time or not—I can enjoy it in a controlled manner and simply don't crave it as often. Nowadays, I am amazed those same commercials and pictures of sugar cookie dough barely get a reaction out of me. When I consider the prison cell of food addiction I lived in for most of my life, this is nothing short of a miracle.

Chapter 9 Take-Home Messages

✓Make every calorie count by only eating things you enjoy.

✓Take the time to figure out foods that you love and foods that you like. Try to only spend calories on foods you love or those with nutritional value.

✓Learn to differentiate between the two kinds of desires involved in eating: Mr. Right-Now desire vs. Mr. Right desire.

✓The satisfaction we get from food doesn't increase as we get full, but diminishes with every bite.

✓If you train your mind into experiencing closure in all things you eat, you will consume fewer calories, resulting in faster weight loss.

✓Take the food that trips you up and cut the recipe or portions down to the appropriate size.

✓Remove temptation. Quit worrying about food going to waste and learn to be okay with throwing out food that is going to your waist.

✓Because we eat healthy and smart for non-eventful meals, we don't feel guilty for the occasional splurge or feast when traveling. Restaurants do not need to be a landmine. Plan ahead and use closure to your advantage.

✓Don't let special moments pass you by. Avoid wasting your calories by eating only what you really enjoy. Above all, follow peace!

You Reap What You Sow

You'll never change your life until you change something you do daily. The secret of your success is found in your daily routine.
~John C. Maxwell

Lara

The other day, as I was getting my haircut, my stylist made a great observation. She said, "You know, it isn't like my body became out of shape overnight. It happened little by little over the course of several months and eventually turned to a body I didn't like any more." We discussed how easy it was to assume one small poor decision on a daily basis can be so harmless. It seemed insignificant at the time, but when you reflect over a course of a year, it is mind-blowing the repercussions caused by all of those little decisions.

I can think of numerous times I failed to make smart food choices before I had peace in this area. Instead of giving these choices the attention they deserved, I would quickly tell myself I would try better tomorrow and continue throwing more food in my mouth. Tomorrow would come and go, and the outcome would continue to be negative. Here is the kicker that I didn't realize:

Failure to choose = Choosing results I didn't want

Who would actually choose bad health, an overweight body, low energy, low quality of life, and poor self-confidence? When you hesitate or fail to take action, those results are exactly what you've chosen.

Most people with bad eating habits along with inactive lifestyles didn't set out to be unhealthy. Instead, they most likely put off what they know they should do. They have good intentions, but instead, are getting exactly what they don't want.

It is a life law that you reap what you sow. Keep sowing those seeds day in and day out, and eventually you will reap a harvest. Yes, even hesitation and waiting is a seed you sow, with results you don't want. So, if you've been waiting for the push to finally get headed in the right direction, consider this: When you close this book and continue through your day, you'll be planting a seed. Will the one you plant bring a plentiful harvest or a field of weeds? One of these is inevitable because harvest time is coming. So choose wisely.

This chapter is devoted to taking all the knowledge you have gathered thus far and putting it into action. Let's start sowing those seeds!

Self-Control

"A person without self-control is like a city with broken-down walls."
~Proverbs 25:28 (NLT)

In ancient times, cities were built with walls around them for one main purpose—protection. Their walls acted as a defense from intruders and outsiders. It allowed them to regulate who they allowed in and out.

You too have a similar wall that can protect you. That wall is self-control. For some people, their walls are broken down by the lack of self-control and, as a result, their lives are filled with chaos.

However, for the person who has developed and maintained self-control, there is a protection around their life as it keeps the good in and the bad out.

Self-control is one of the defining differences you will find between a successful and an unsuccessful person: self-control in their thoughts, what they chose to believe, their habits, and their actions. If you desire success, you'll need this quality.

Start building your wall of protection. It takes only one brick at a time to eventually create a wall of strength.

Habits

Successful people are simply those with successful habits.
~Brian Tracy

Robynn
"You'll never get down to your optimal weight."
"It's just too hard to lose the weight."
"Just throw in the towel today, eat whatever you want, and start over tomorrow."

These are some of the phrases that have cycled through my mind hundreds, if not thousands of times throughout my life. Over time, these thoughts became a negative habit determining the course of my life. Thankfully, when I began my journey, I slowly developed habits that served the purpose of reaching my goals.

Habits are probably the single most important factor affecting your level of peace with your body, weight, exercise, and food. And for the majority of people, habits will determine whether you are at the optimal weight zone for your body frame, musculature, metabolism, and build. Because, like it or not, habits are what chart the course of our life. If you trace the life of a truly successful person, you will find they are tethered to a string of habits that support their successful life. And conversely, if you trace the life of an unsuccessful person, you will find they are tethered to habits that lead to an unsuccessful life.

In fact, we can take it a step further and say each area of our life, successful or unsuccessful, is tied to habits. Our goal regarding this book is to identify and develop the habits that will lead to peace with your body, weight, exercise, and food. Once we do, the rest falls into place.

When I was a teacher, brain research was an extremely popular topic. Although I have been out of education for close to a decade, I'm guessing such data is still highly valuable information. After all, if we want students to succeed and maximize their potential, it is imperative that a teacher understands how the learning process occurs and then implement it in teaching.

One fascinating thing brain research has shown is how deeply ingrained habits are formed. From research, we see that neurons in our brain form pathways or tunnels each time we do something new. As these new behaviors are repeated, the pathway is established and the habit becomes ingrained. Once the habit is ingrained, the neurons automatically travel down this pathway. It is sort of like digging a tunnel. At first the work is long and tedious, but after the tunnel is dug you can easily pass through.

Remember back to how awkward learning to drive a car was. The whole process of talking to yourself step-by-step, saying, "Ok, put your left foot on the brake. Oops, I mean the right foot on the brake. Then put the car in reverse. Now put your foot on the accelerator. Oops! Forgot to *gently* put my right foot on the accelerator..." However, within a few months, driving a car becomes old hat. You don't think about which foot to place on the accelerator or when to turn on your blinker. You simply do it because in your brain a pathway for this behavior has been created.

It is in these situations that habits work to our advantage. They free our minds and allow us to expend our mental energy on things that need our focus and attention.

However, bad habits work the same way. They are ingrained and automatic, so much so that you probably don't even realize what you are doing.

Maybe when you were a child, you developed the habit of turning to food every time you experienced uncomfortable feelings and negative emotions. It might be that you didn't have the emotional or physical support you needed, so instead of turning to unreliable and unavailable people, you turned to food.

Or flash back to your college days. Perhaps you picked up some habits that packed on the pounds and/or sent you down a path of unhealthy habits.

We all have habits that aren't serving our best interests and changing them is harder than it sounds. After all, there is a reason why only eleven percent of people actually fulfill their New Year's resolutions.

We'll tackle how to break a bad habit in the next vignette, but for now remember this: Your habits will determine your outcomes.

Lara: In the past, I associated the word "habits" with something bad. Now I've realized how habits are a good thing when creating ones that work to your advantage. After applying a tool, such as identifying a Mr. Right food versus a Mr. Right-Now food, good habits have saved me from wasting a lot of excess calories. Good habits are now so automatic it takes very little thought, and I naturally make smarter decisions!

Redirect Bad Habits

*Your net worth to the world is usually determined by what
remains after your bad habits are subtracted from your good
ones.*
~Benjamin Franklin

Robynn

Unfortunately, once a bad habit is created in your brain, it can't
be broken because pathways reinforcing this habit have been
created, and they are there for life. But the redeeming news is that
you can create a new habit that routes a different pathway.

This reminds me of going to an indoor water park with my kids
and husband. My six-year-old talked me into going down the big
loop-de-loop slide that was about three or four stories tall. At the
top of the stairs, there was not one, but two slides. One was pitch-
black. The other slide allowed light through its blue plastic tube. Of
course, the slide my daughter wanted to go down was pitch-dark. I
obliged her once, but being in a totally dark slide for five to ten
seconds was enough for me!

After that experience, I realized how similar these two slides are
to the habits we form. If you've developed a dark habit, the good
news is you can form a new habit that brings light and peace to
your life. The tunnel to the old, dark habit will remain, but each
time you get to the top of those stairs, you get to decide which
pathway to take.

For example, if you have a bad habit of overeating at office
parties, you may think eliminating all meals with co-workers is
necessary. It's easy to get caught up in the all-or-nothing approach.
However, let's say the problem is piling huge servings on your
plate and going back for seconds. Creating a new habit of taking
small servings of your favorite foods and avoiding seconds may
take time. Rest assured, before too long you can enjoy your
coworkers and comfort foods without overeating.

Think about when you get tripped up in your eating or where
you lack peace with food. Maybe ninety-five percent of the time
you experience happiness, but the other five percent is spent
dealing with uncomfortable, defeating, or tumultuous feelings.

Don't underestimate even the small five percent. Regardless of how minor those issues may seem, deal with them today and begin heading down the right path.

Lara: Eating while I prepared meals was a habit I struggled with for years. If I was gathering the ingredients for spaghetti in the pantry and saw chips or candy on the shelf, I would grab and munch on them as I made dinner. By the time we sat down to eat, I would be full. Unfortunately, that didn't stop me from also eating the meal I'd spent thirty minutes preparing. Over time I have changed that habit by chewing gum, brushing my teeth, or putting on whitening strips before cooking. Doing so distracts me from wanting to put something in my mouth and allows me to fully enjoy mealtime because I am hungry when I sit down to eat.

Robynn: A bad habit I changed was going to Subway and getting a Subway Melt, Sun Chips, diet pop, and three cookies. I didn't need to quit going to Subway. I just needed to replace my bad habit with a good one. Now I get a kid's meal—sandwich with veggies, Baked Lays, and water. It took a little while to make this a habit, but now it is my new norm. Another habit I formed (which has taken a lot of practice and time) was to stop grazing. I used to eat a little bite here and there, between meals all day long. Grazing is one thing that leads me to eating an excessive amount of extra calories. When afternoon hunger or the urge to eat strikes, I go for fruit. It's healthy, doesn't give me a lot of unnecessary calories, and most importantly

never leads to the throw-in-the-towel mindset
that causes me to go on an all-out binge.

Substitute Bad Habits with Good Ones

If you go to a tree with an ax and take five whacks at the tree
every day, it doesn't matter if it's an oak or a redwood;
eventually the tree has to fall down.
~Jack Canfield

We've been talking about negative habits and how to replace them with productive ones. Maybe you have so many habits you want to change that you are at a loss over where to start.

We are both fans of money-management expert Dave Ramsey's approach to getting out of debt. He calls it the Debt Snowball. This is a technique where you list all your debts from least to greatest, and you begin chipping away at reducing those debts by paying off the smallest debt first. This way, with every effort, you begin to see the snowball effect of debt reduction.

Peace with food has a similar concept for reducing bad habits. Begin by prioritizing the habits you want to change. For example, if your biggest weakness is portion control, write it at the top of your list. After compiling your list, begin substituting a new habit for the old one you want to change. To help with portion control, dish up your plate first and put the rest away in the fridge. Don't worry about how long it takes to get a new habit established. Some may take a few weeks, others a few months, but focusing on one habit at a time will ultimately result in progress toward your goal.

Once a new habit is in place, begin with the next habit on your list. It won't be long before you begin to see positive changes and gain confidence.

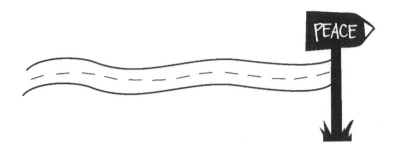

T. Changing Lane Signs

Your Habits—What bad habits can you break by creating new ones?

Negative Habit	New Habit

Lara

Negative Habit	New Habit
Wasting calories on food I don't love.	Spend calories only on food I love or what my body needs.
Feeling guilty because I ate something I love—chocolate chip cookies.	Giving myself permission to enjoy cookies in a controlled manner.
Eating off my kids' plates when cleaning off the table.	Make my kids dump their food in the trash and clear their plates as soon as they are done eating.
Feeling the need to finish off a row of brownies.	Throw out or give away the rest of the dessert.
Overeating takeout food.	Dish out the food on plates and put the leftovers in the fridge before we sit down to eat.

Robynn

Negative Habit	New Habit
Grazing all day in the pantry.	Eliminate grazing. If hungry, choose something I enjoy that also benefits me nutritionally.
Having tempting foods in the house.	Keep tempting foods out of house. If I give myself permission to have tempting food, eat a pre-determined amount and remove the rest.
Volunteering to bake for other people on unique occasions (baby shower, funeral, etc.).	Baking presents too many temptations. Instead, buy prepackaged foods or volunteer for a different task.
Spending days trying to get back on track after I ate much more than I had planned.	Avoid the throw-in-the-towel mindset by hitting reset after eating more than I had planned.
Eating all my calories in the morning and then feeling deprived when I can't eat dinner with my family.	Spread out my calories throughout the day. Save sufficient amount of calories for dinner so I don't feel deprived.

Make Adjustments Then Try Again

*It's fine to celebrate success but it is more important to heed the
lessons of failure.*
~Bill Gates

Robynn

Krispy Kreme® donuts. Yum. My mouth begins watering just
thinking about them. There was a time where they pulled me in
hook, line, and sinker.

I thought in order to enjoy the full Krispy Kreme®
experience, I had to buy a dozen. Not one donut, not two, but a
dozen. After all, I live over two hours from the nearest location,
and who knows when I will get this opportunity again?

After consuming the lion's share of the dozen, I would
inevitably feel miserable. I knew there had to be a better way.
There had to be a way I could enjoy these donuts and have
peace. Eventually I trained myself to buy one or two, savor
every bite, and then say "Ciao!"

This isn't rocket science, but before my journey, I would not
have tried to find peace with Krispy Kreme® donuts. I've
learned that taking all of my favorite foods through this process
is important, even if it means I crash and burn before finding an
alternative that brings peace.

After years of dieting, eating in a way that gives true
satisfaction and freedom may seem foreign to you. In fact,
without a regimen of restrictive rules and food lists, you may be
at a loss. You are being empowered to create your own
customized lifestyle, but this idea scares you. The good news is,
you don't have to do it alone. To help you succeed, you have a
handful of resources, including your posse and Posse Partner (if
you choose to enlist their help) along with the tools in this book.
But maybe best of all, you have a teacher—and this teacher's
name is *Failure*.

First of all, we can't ever consider failure as negative. That's
because your greatest successes will be hidden within the
lessons taught to you by this great teacher. And as with most
great teachers, you usually don't appreciate them until after

learning their lessons. It's when you are down the road and their invaluable lessons prove to be beneficial that you are grateful you were their student.

The best way to respond to failure so you can learn the lesson quickly and with the least pain possible is by adjusting and reattempting. The process looks like this:

Educated Attempt→Fail→Adjust→Reattempt

Simply give it your best shot, and if your attempt fails, take note, make adjustments, and try again, this time wiser than before. Eventually, you'll find what works. Once you do, the process looks like this:

Educated Attempt→Succeed→Repeat

In this way, failure is responsible for educating you in what works and what doesn't. In fact, we believe the best way to find out what works is by finding out what doesn't.

So don't be afraid of failure. Do your homework, seek all the wisdom you can, and then it's time to jump in with both feet. Your greatest successes may be hidden within your greatest failures. Don't be afraid of them. They may be the best teacher you've ever had.

Lara: My teacher named Failure has taught me a lot. Through my journey, I learned that when daily events stressed me out, I would shut my mind off out of frustration and grab whatever food was available at the time. I learned that I used my stress as an excuse to "act" like I was unaware of my poor eating choices, although deep down I was fully conscience of my actions. After many attempts and adjustments, I can now say that I no longer struggle in this area. I can now identify when I am overwhelmed and handle it successfully without using food as a coping method.

Overcome Temptation

To be prepared for war is one of the most effective means of
preserving peace.
~George Washington

Life is good. You've been eating well for days. You're feeling great, and the number on the scale continues to fall. You're certain this is it; you are *finally* going to lose the weight for good. Then, out of nowhere, a temptation whacks you over the head. What seemed to be an ironclad amount of self-control instantly becomes a full-fledged eating spree.

We can be so blindsided with temptation. Things can be going so smoothly, and suddenly we find ourselves spiraling out of control. If you have had this experience, you no doubt understand the ensuing frustration, discouragement, and despair.

If temptation was an unpredictable phenomenon with no way to prepare or plan ahead, we would have an excuse for feeling helpless. We would be the slaves of this ruthless master with no hope of redemption. But the liberating truth is we don't have to be victims of our impulses and urges. We can learn how and when temptation works and be prepared to meet it head-on.

Let's talk about what temptation is and how it works.

The What: Temptation is an extremely appealing call to do something we know we shouldn't due to legal or moral reasons. A temptation gives the impression of being insurmountable and unrelenting. Because of its intimidating nature, many times it causes its victims to surrender in defeat without a fight. But as overwhelming as temptation may seem, its power is deceptive and short-lived. This is precisely why we must learn to handle it appropriately and immediately.

Although two people may be challenged in similar areas, their level of receptiveness and ability to deal with these challenges will differ. Each person also has different catalysts that trigger them to overeat, such as social settings, time of day, or mood.

No one is immune to temptation. It is a fact of life. If you feel like a helpless victim, be encouraged. You can become skillful at successfully handling it. Here's how.

The How: To overcome temptation, you must understand how it works. We like to compare it to going off a high dive at a swimming pool. Before you take the final step that sends you free falling, you have to climb a ladder and then take a handful of steps to the end of the board. With each rung of the ladder and each step on the board, you become more committed to jumping off the high dive. Changing your mind isn't a big deal after taking the first step up the ladder. But by the time you are on the end of the board, it is difficult (but not impossible) to go back. Once you take that last step off the board, there is no turning back. Regardless of how badly you want to change your mind as you are accelerating 9.8m/s^2 to the water, gravity is king.

When it comes to temptation, there is a point at which "gravity" will take over. Regardless of how much you wish you weren't falling, the decision has already been made. If you want to increase your success at overcoming temptation, your mission is to cut out the preliminary steps leading up to the final fall. After all, it's impossible to go off the ten-foot high dive if you never take the steps to climb the ladder and walk to the end of the board. The best news of all is that the easiest way to overcome the string of temptation is to stop at the first step.

It's interesting to note that the first step of temptation usually occurs in your mind with a suggestive thought. You may be minding your own business when a temptation is presented to you. Let's say you see a television commercial for a greasy bacon cheeseburger and fries. Immediately you think about heading to the nearest fast-food joint. If you don't nix that thought immediately, you are taking step one. Practice eliminating this step. We say practice because you won't do this thing perfectly. Over time, if you are diligent, you will see improvement. And one last thing: for best results remember you can always utilize help from God.

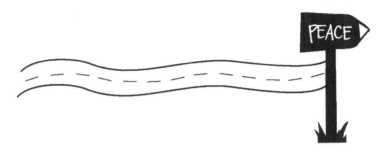

U. Rocky Cliffs

Temptation—What trips you up? (Food, situations, people, emotions, and time of day.)

In the table below, list the temptations that trip you up along with the first step of the temptation solution.

Temptation	How To Deal With It
Ex: Buying an excess of junk food at the grocery store.	Ex. Make a grocery list and stick only to the list.

Lara (before peace with food): Seconds and eating off kids' plates, any type of home baked dessert on the counter, and Puppy Chow during the holidays.

Lara (after peace with food): If I get lazy and (1) don't make my kids clean their own plates after a meal and (2) don't create closure with my desserts and snacks.

Robynn (before peace with food): Cookie dough, having more than one helping of home cooked food, banana nut bread hot out of the oven, over eating at meals that aren't regular events, such as Thanksgiving. Once a year pancake feed.

Robynn (after peace with food): I now understand that food is no longer the issue. Instead, the things that can trip me up now are: not having closure; panicking because I'm focused on my weight and not on developing character; discouragement; and any time I begin taking on a diet mentality, something in me always rebels.

Let Wisdom Do the Heavy Lifting

Do for yourself when you're strong what you can't do when you're weak.
~Willie George

Robynn
Boy oh boy, have I ever been blindsided by temptation. There were times when I said something I knew I would regret and later had to humble myself and apologize. Other times, I got myself into tempting situations and was luckily able to escape by the skin of my teeth. Someone please remind me never to do that again!

Eliminating temptation when it first appears on your doorstep is good, but preparing for it before it shows up is even better. The best way to do this is to know your internal clock. Ask yourself, "When are you most vulnerable to temptation? Is it early in the morning, when you are watching television, cooking dinner?" You have to know when you are most susceptible and make provisions to remove yourself from that situation.

It is easy to think when things are going well that we are resistant to temptation. This is a flat out lie! You can use your moments of strength to prepare for times when darts are hurled your way. An example would include removing food that has tripped you up in the past that will be a trigger when you're feeling weak in the future.

The foods you need to be most wary of are the right-now foods—foods you don't love but eat because they are accessible. If we are not careful, moments of weakness will cause us to eat even though we don't really desire them. To be successful, we do our best to avoid having these foods easily available. Keeping them out of sight and out of mind helps rid us of this type of mindless eating.

Another way you can use your moments of strength to prepare for temptation is when you go shopping. Let's say you are buying groceries and walk past the donut aisle. Although you had no intention of buying donuts, you are tempted, even though you know it is not a good idea. You throw them in the cart, pay for them, and take them home. At this point, the chances that you won't dive in are not very good!

So many times we try to stop this free fall after we're already at the very end of the diving board. It's crazy to think we do this to ourselves, yet we do it all the time. We talk a lot about stopping the insane cycle, and this is one of those cycles.

If you are serious about stopping your temptations, you must do this at the first step rather than the last. The first step is the easiest place to stop the free fall because the temptation has not picked up momentum. It isn't rocket science, it's called wisdom.

Next time you are in the grocery store and the box of donuts is begging to jump in your cart, you have a decision to make. All it takes is walking away, and immediately the temptation is gone. You just let wisdom—the sense to know the temptation is short-lived—do the heavy lifting.

Lara: When I plan ahead, for example, I can have my premade energy balls for breakfast so I know what to eat each morning. If I get lazy and don't make a batch before I run out, I have learned I turn to sugary pre-packaged breakfast snacks that will later leave me hungry and sluggish. Not only that, it usually results in poor eating the rest of the day because I started the morning on the wrong foot.

Be Prepared for a Temptation

Part of the happiness of life consists not in fighting battles, but in avoiding them. A masterly retreat is in itself a victory.
~Norman Vincent Peale

We wish we could tell you there will come a time when you will be immune to temptation, but we can't. Temptation is a part of life. Instead of spending your time hoping it won't attack you, you have to prepare yourself by being armed and ready.

You can handle this situation by realizing that, as painful as your temptation may be, it is short-lived. It is similar to a huge ocean wave that gains speed and height and then crests. Your temptation will crest, and until it does, hang on! Don't let it overtake you.

Engage in an activity that will get your mind off of the temptation. Use some of these strategies or come up with your own:

- Get Out of Dodge! If possible, get away from the point of your temptation. Most likely, if you are at home, your temptation will be in the kitchen. If so, move to another part of your house, play with your kids in their playroom, tackle cleaning out a closet, or head outdoors.
- Grab your keys and go for a drive. Many times we eat because we are bored or feel pressure. Could the pressure be from needy children? Driving can be comforting for both you and your kids. A change of scenery may be all you need. Maybe you'll even end up at the park and get some exercise.
- Do something food related that doesn't take up calories. Chew gum, drink water, or munch on veggies.

You must fill your time with something. Don't just sit around thinking about resisting the temptation because, chances are, you will give in to the temptation. Instead, consider doing something productive. Find activities that are:

- **Necessary**—Run errands you've been putting off.
- **Enjoyable**—Call a friend.
- **Relaxing**—Take a bath.
- **Taxing, But Rewarding**—Engage in physical or mental activities like household chores, exercise, or reading.

When temptation comes knocking, you don't have to invite it in and entertain it. Instead, be prepared to send that unwelcome guest on its way.

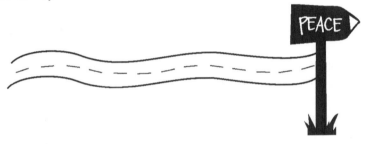

V. Surfboard Shop
Outlasting the Temptation Waves—What strategies will help you outlast the temptation wave?

- _____
- _____
- _____
- _____
- _____
- _____
- _____

Lara and Robynn: We both run out the clock (see next vignette) by getting busy doing something that will distract our thoughts. We know the wave will eventually subside so we

are determined to outlast the temptation. We
also ask God for help or call a Posse
Partner.

Use Procrastination to Your Advantage

There aren't too many times in life when procrastination is a good
thing, but in the game of basketball, as well as in peace with food,
procrastination can be a lifesaver. If you've ever watched
basketball, you know that "running out the clock" means the
leading team basically plays keep-away from their opponent until
the end of the game.

We call this technique using procrastination to your advantage,
and here is when you use it: you want to eat, but don't know what.
When you find yourself in this predicament, it is a sure sign you
want to eat for reasons other than having a legitimate desire for
food. Maybe you're bored, stressed, or feeling ambiguous, not
knowing what it is you want in life. Or maybe you are tempted to
eat something you know you shouldn't. It is in these moments that
running out the clock is our strategy.

The reason it works so well is that these moments, as in a
basketball game, don't go on forever. Usually these feelings last
only a short time, therefore, outlasting them can help you win the
game.

So the next time you find yourself at the refrigerator staring at
the contents for something that sounds good to eat, understand the
opponent you're facing. It's times like these when we need to call a
time-out and a play that runs out the clock. That may mean calling
a friend, going for a walk, or getting busy. The game doesn't last
forever, so beat the opponent by running out the clock.

Rip It like a Band-Aid® and Build Momentum

Inaction breeds doubt and fear. Action breeds confidence and courage. If you want to conquer fear, do not sit home and think about it. Go out and get busy.
~Dale Carnegie

Lara

I don't know about you, but even though all this peace with food stuff works on most days, some days I still have a hard time mustering up the energy when I'm feeling sluggish or in a funk. Maybe you've been eating great, working out, and trying your best to stay positive, but emotionally you just can't kick it. Or maybe having a rough day is causing you to lose peace, resulting in out-of-control eating. In these moments we suggest you rip it like a Band-Aid®.

You have to engage your body to disengage your brain. No putting it off, no over thinking it. Just do what you need to do—right now! Get it over with, the way you rip off a bandage. Come on. Ripping it off isn't nearly as painful as the anticipation of doing something you are dreading. Stop thinking about it and just do it!

By being productive, you can increase your chances of reversing the funk because you build positive momentum and get traction under your belt.

I rarely look forward to working out. Believe me when I say that talking myself into exercising, whether I'm in a funk or not, takes a lot of work. But when I remember to get in the "rip it" mindset, it makes all the difference in the world. I turn my mind off by avoiding thoughts of how much I am dreading the workout. Instead, I just rip it and do it. And when I'm done I feel like I can take on the world. (Okay, not really the world, but it sure does seem to motivate me the rest of the day.)

Some days are extra challenging because I feel like I have to rip it all day long in order to avoid letting the bad feelings take over my day. When this happens, you have to remind yourself this experience is common. Just ride it out. Keep trying different methods to fight the funk, and soon it will be over.

Don't let your emotions pull you down another day. Rip it like a Band-Aid®. Rest assured, it will only sting for a second.

Prepare for a Bad Day

There are many ways you can deal with the funk. We've tried to give you numerous methods for dealing with these negative emotions, but ultimately, you'll have to determine what works best for you. As with every other aspect of your journey, this will take practice. Use what has worked in the past and try some new approaches.

To get you started, here are a few examples:

- Call your Posse Partner.
- Rip it like a Band-Aid® by getting busy doing something productive.
- Take a look at your goals.

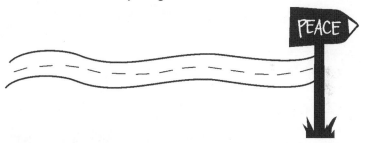

W. Lifeguard Stand
Survival Kit—What items are in your survival kit to get you through challenging times?

- _____
- _____
- _____
- _____
- _____
- _____
- _____

Lara: Redirect my thoughts by getting busy, burning a candle to make my house smell fresh, or call Robynn for encouragement.

Robynn: A phone call to Lara, uplifting and encouraging music, motivational and inspiring CD's, being productive and getting my mind off of food, reflecting on my vision board, looking at my goals and speaking positive affirmations, and encouraging myself that this challenge is temporary, but the character growth gained will be permanent.

Be Flexible and Adaptable

Enjoying success requires the ability to adapt. Only by being open to change will you have a true opportunity to get the most from your talent.
~Nolan Ryan

Lara

I do not like to weigh in every day. For some reason, it causes me to feel like I'm controlled by the scale. As an experiment for this book, I tried to weigh in daily and document how my new exercise regimen affected my weight. After about three weeks, I could see the scale caused me to cut back immensely on my food intake due to stressing about the next weigh-in. Since the anxiety already skewed my results, I had to tweak the experiment by weighing in on a two-week basis instead of every day. I was able to get more accurate results (even though it was every two weeks) because the stress of daily weigh-ins was no longer an issue.

To have continual peace, you will have to be flexible. Your circumstances in life will always change and you will need to adjust your eating and exercise to guarantee you don't lose peace. Your ability to adapt will determine your success.

Let's say you love to run, but you get injured. If you want to continue to work out until you are healed enough to run again, you will have to be open to other forms of exercise. If the idea of doing a one-hour workout video doesn't bring you happiness, walking in place during your favorite television program may be the alternative. Remaining happy and active is what peace is all about.

So always remember, you will have to periodically adapt to your season of life because circumstances are never constant.

Document Your Progress

Writing down bits and pieces of your journey can be beneficial because it gives you a snapshot of significant points along the way. Sort of like the snapshots you take on a vacation—tracking moments that would otherwise be forgotten.

Tracking may sound time consuming, but it actually can be as simple as checks or marks on a calendar. The information is invaluable because it allows you to determine cause and effect and then proceed smarter, wiser, and armed with knowledge. Tracking allows you to connect the dots so you can set yourself up for success. It helps you understand *you* better.

If you are new at tracking, you'll have to determine what is most important and helpful because, as we say, there is no one-size-fits-all way to do it. Here are some things you could track:

- **Rate Your Level of Peace**—On a scale from zero to five, track your peace each day or week. If your number goes down, evaluate why. You may need to make adjustments or see if it was based on a mood you were in. If the number goes up, evaluate why and keep doing it.
- **Weigh on a Regular Basis**—Weekly or monthly.
- **Measurements**—On a monthly basis, track things such as waist, hips, bust, thighs, and arms. You can also measure BMI, % fat, and % muscle, if you have a scale with that option.
- **Food Consumption**—What you eat and how much.
- **Emotions**—Do emotions trigger you to overeat? If so, what was the emotion? Why were you feeling that way? What time of the month were you feeling this way? (Maybe you get stressed at the end of the month

paycheck wise. Also, women may experience emotional ups and downs monthly. This information can help you come up with a plan for these occasions.)

• **What Trips You Up**—Situations, people, times of day, emotions, and triggers such as food commercials.
• **Exercise**—What type of activity and when.

As we said, you may decide some of these areas of tracking are helpful, or you may not find them useful at all. Lara tracks her weight whenever she feels like it, usually a couple times a month. She also makes notes of her emotions on occasion. Robynn, on the other hand, is obsessed with tracking! She writes down her weight weekly, and from time to time, she records her BMI, % fat, % weight, exercise (when and what she did), and what she eats.

That's what we track. Now it's your turn to take action. Grab your journal, iPhone, graphing paper, calendar—whatever is most beneficial for you—and start jotting down the clues that will help you discover your way to peace.

Utilize Your Resources

Do what you can, with what you have, where you are.
~Theodore Roosevelt

Lara

Running shoes. Check.
Treadmill. Check.
Motivation. Check.
One mile down, one mile to go. Check.

Yep, I was feelin' pretty good. I committed to walking on the treadmill two miles a day, and I had a handful of successes under my belt. Life is pretty easy when everything works in my favor.

But let's face it. It is pretty rare that you can *check, check, check,* and not have a single hang-up.

As I said, I was one mile down, one mile to go. I was golden. Then it happened. My son, who was doing such a great job playing on his own, tripped and fell, resulting in sobs and a need to be consoled.

I glanced at the treadmill screen. Only 0.4 miles. Should I let him cry it out? *I can't believe I just thought that! I'm such a terrible mother. He needs me!* Okay, what will bring me peace? I can either pitch the all-or-nothing mindset and be happy with the 1.6 miles, or I can use the resources I have and finish this puppy out.

So I grabbed my little guy, wiped his tears, held him, and I walked. That's right. I walked slowly on the treadmill for the last 0.4 miles. Running would have been challenging (and dangerous!), but by walking, I was able to soothe him and finish what I started.

Sometimes we have to use the resources readily available to get the job done. I wish life always worked the way I map it out in my mind, but the majority of the time, it doesn't. Instead of using this as an excuse never to start something, but instead accept the fact that I will have curve balls, I am mentally prepared to adapt and utilize resources I have.

What things are you not doing because you are worried they won't go as planned? Can you just start and make the adjustments as challenges arise?

In a perfect world, we would be living with a perfect body, in a perfect environment, with a perfect life. But we don't live in a perfect world. Each of us is dealt a unique set of circumstances, along with the challenge to take what we've been given and make the best of it.

Maybe your resources are few and far between. Maybe they are anything but ideal. Even so, don't despise the limited resources you do have, instead, use them to your advantage. Once you do, you'll find they begin to multiply.

What are your resources? It's easy to think only of money, education, or position, but don't discount some of the following:

- **Time**—Since your Tuesday nights are free and you've wanted to meet new people, why not sign up for water aerobics?
- **Childcare**—Do you have someone who could watch your kids a few hours a week while you work out? Could you take turns with a friend watching their kids, then them watching yours?

- **Relationships/Connections**—Do you know someone who is already a shoe-in to be your Posse Partner?
- **Personality**—Do you have a personality trait that loves to get in front of people? Maybe it could be utilized by training to lead Jazzercise classes.
- **House/Space**—We have a friend who bought a home in the country with a shed on the property. When she lived in the city, she was a fitness instructor. Now she uses the shed to her advantage by offering fitness classes there. With all the space, moms can exercise while their kids ride bikes, play, and have a good time.
- **Passion**—What do you love doing? How could you incorporate that into a healthy lifestyle?
- **Family and Friends**—What individuals can you turn to when dealing with a food temptation? How can you distract your thoughts?
- **Ideas**—What ideas are floating around in your head? Is it a new strategy for your journey? If so, give it a try and see if it works. If it doesn't meet your expectations then view it as a lesson learned, not a failure.

Reach your goals in regards to eating and exercise by utilizing the resources right at your fingertips.

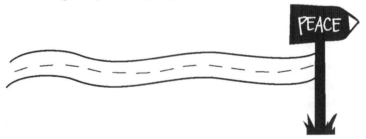

X. Backpack
Your Resources—What resources can help you live at peace with food?

- _____
- _____
- _____

- _____
- _____
- _____
- _____

Lara: I love doing projects at home, and if I can pick up my pace while doing them, I can burn the same calories I would on the treadmill. I can also do household chores at a faster speed, which gets my heart rate up and makes me more efficient with my tasks around the house.

Robynn: Utilizing grandparents so I can go running or walking.

Develop Skills for Success

Success is a science; if you have the conditions, you get the result.
~Oscar Wilde

Robynn

Have you ever watched a mystery movie that kept you on the edge of your seat until the secrets were revealed in the end? In a really good mystery, you never figure it out until this climatic moment. This takes me back to my childhood when my dad would buy my mom the big heart-shaped box of chocolates. You never knew what type of chocolate you were getting and, as a result, you tried a lot of chocolates until you found the one you actually liked.

Some have a misconception that success is like that heart-shaped box of chocolates. They think it is a total mystery. This flawed mindset assumes people are successful because they are lucky or were at the right place at the right time.

But that is not the way life works. Although our world is constantly changing, life is actually quite predictable. That's because there is a science to how things work. Sure, luck can play a part in someone's success, and sometimes the world seems to get turned upside down due to unexpected events. But even then, successful people know how to make things—good or bad—work to their advantage. There is a science to success, and truly successful people have this science mastered.

Take a look at successful people, and you will find a common denominator—they are skillful in what matters most in their area of expertise. They consistently perform at the top of their game.

Skillful people know the tools they need and use them to their advantage to achieve their desired outcome. Although there are general tools to success, such as wisdom, hard work, and commitment, the tools you require will be unique to you. To be successful you must determine which tools can help reach your goals.

Think of all the people who are master craftsmen in their field. They each have special tools. A carpenter would use a hammer and saw, whereas a speaker would use storytelling and an inviting stage presence. If you took the tools away from these individuals, they would cease to be skillful in their area of expertise.

Peace with food is no different. To be a master of your craft you will need tools to help you acquire skills. In this chapter, we gave tools to help you with habits, temptation, and moments of weakness, but you'll need to determine which ones work for you. And among the ones that work, some will be more effective or simply more preferred than others.

A thought to ponder: If you are struggling with your weight or lack of peace with your body and/or food, it is not because you are inadequate or flawed. Rather, you simply do not have the skills you need. At least, not yet.

It's similar to the learning that takes place in school. A kindergartener is not expected to have the skills of a high school senior. Although the kindergartener can succeed at her present level, she has much more to learn.

No matter what your level, you can make forward progress. So let's get rollin'. In the upcoming rest stop, you will record the tools you'll need. If you want help getting started, we included a list with some of the tools we use.

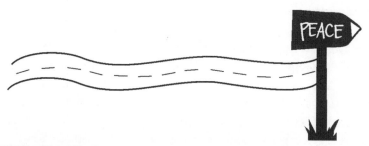

Y. The Tool Store

Tools needed to help you succeed—What tools do you need to help you become skillful at having peace with food and your body? Examples include:

- A posse
- This book
- Scale that records weight, BMI, % body fat, % muscle
- Motivational music, books, DVDs and CDs
- Walking path
- Apps to help count calories/points, track exercise, or plan meals
- Bike, treadmill, or other exercise equipment
- Fitness class or running club
- Activity tracker to wear throughout the day

List your tools below. The sky is the limit, so be creative!

- _____
- _____
- _____
- _____
- _____
- _____
- _____

Lara: Reading a few vignettes of this book whenever I am having an "off" day, talking to Robynn, jotting down my weight a few times a month, and wearing my Fitbit® activity tracker daily.

Robynn: Frequent talks with Lara; a scale that measures BMI, body percent fat and muscle; Weight Watchers® meetings and online tools; biking path in the warmer months and treadmill in the colder months; my vision board; written out positive affirmations and goals; motivating/inspiring books; and last but not least, prayer.

Lara and Robynn: Remember, when we set out to find peace with food, we had no idea whether or not we would figure it out—or how. All we knew was we never wanted to diet again, and there had to be a better approach to food. The most important tool we had at the time was each other. We knew if we talked through our experiences and how we were feeling, we would eventually discover the answer. Looking back, we are glad we didn't underestimate the power of this tool. With each other's support, we became skillful at finding the outcome we had been longing for: peace!

Make a Plan and Start Today

If you go to work on your goals, your goals will go to work on you. If you go to work on your plan, your plan will go to work on you. Whatever good things we build end up building us.
~Jim Rohn

Robynn
The Brooklyn Bridge and forty-degree rainy weather. That was the setting on April 5, 2003, when Scott proposed to me. This famous bridge then became part of our history. Its iconic symbolism also became the theme behind our wedding. Wedding

gifts, reception murals, and party favors bore images of this landmark.

One of my favorite pictures of the Brooklyn Bridge is a blueprint replica that hangs in our entryway. It looks like the original that the architect, John A. Roebling, might have drawn up himself.

Although my picture is not the actual Brooklyn Bridge, it is a blueprint of what the bridge looks like. And as with all blueprints, it was created before the structure it represents.

The same is true for living a life of peace with food. It doesn't just happen. It doesn't fall out of the sky and pleasantly surprise you. It is planned. It is specific. It comes by design and not by accident.

In his book, *The 7 Habits of Highly Effective People*, Stephen Covey shares the importance of beginning with the end in mind.[7] This concept is crucial to your success. You cannot mindlessly go throughout life and expect everything to fall right into place. Life does not work that way. Instead, it rewards those who plan intelligently and intentionally and then follows through with those plans.

When constructing your plan, consider the following:

- What is my best-case scenario when it comes to eating?
- What is my acceptable-case scenario when it comes to eating?
- How will a non-eventful/ordinary eating day look?
- How will an out-of-the-ordinary eating day look? What will I do if unexpected dinner plans arise, such as a last-minute invitation from an out-of-town guest?
- What is my plan for exercise? How will I fit it in? What if something comes up? (i.e. You planned to run outdoors, but there is a thunderstorm.)
- How will I eat at my favorite restaurants?
- What is my plan to successfully get through funk days?
- When will I weigh myself after I have a slip-up?

Your plan doesn't have to be perfect. You may even be uncertain about how to start. Don't worry. Just start. With each step, you'll be directed to the next one. You'll start getting a rhythm and things will begin to fall in place. It may not look anything like the original plan but you're making progress and that's the whole point.

Lara: When my husband and I went to Hawaii, I knew I would likely gain weight on the trip because I wanted to enjoy myself in the culture and food. Knowing this, I planned not to weigh myself until one week after returning from the trip. I knew if I saw the inflated weight number on the scale, I would get discouraged. In the past, that discouragement only prolonged my getting back on track with my normal eating. For you, maybe weighing yourself immediately after a trip would be a good reality check and would motivate you to eat well right away. Having a lifestyle tailor made for you will help avoid potential setbacks and discouragement.

Acknowledge Small Steps

The difference between average people and achieving people is their perception of and response to failure.
~John C. Maxwell

Robynn
During our writing process, my family and I vacationed in Colorado. I brought the manuscript to work on during downtime and thought this would be the perfect backdrop for having a clear head and creative mind. I set out on my vacation thinking I would eat moderately as I do on a normal, non-eventful day. However, after having a meal with my family on the first day of the trip, I realized that if I ate as usual, I would be missing out on many of my favorite dining experiences with my loved ones.

My thoughts went immediately to Lara and how she would handle this situation. She has nailed our tool, *Don't Waste Your*

Calories. I, on the other hand, had it mastered on non-eventful days, but on out-of-the-ordinary days, I would usually crash and burn.

I realized I had justified my lack of skill in this principle saying, "It's no big deal. I'll just get back on track after vacation." But after glancing at a draft of our book, I was reminded of our future readers. How could I tell them to do something I wasn't doing?

So on that day, in the middle of my vacation, I made a commitment to acquire the skill of giving myself an inbounds psychological release. I needed to avoid wasting calories and instead only eat in ways that brought me peace. With my all-or-nothing propensity, this would be very challenging. It was my last frontier—the last major skill I lacked. Up to this point, it had been so difficult I pretended it didn't exist. But my bluff had been called, and I would do this no matter how difficult it was.

At the end of the first day of attempting this new skill, I stood in front of the mirror feeling like a total failure. Thoughts even bombarded my mind of aborting this mission. My mind reassured me I could learn this skill later on. And again, I thought about our readers and what I would tell them if they were in my shoes. I looked in that mirror and with great determination said, "I will not quit."

It was time for a reality check. I asked myself, "Did you have any success today? Did you do anything right?" The answer was "Yes." As I recounted the day, I saw that although I had made many mistakes, I did do some things right.

Another realization was that I had always based my feelings of success on whether I thought I had lost weight. It was time for me to replace that question with a much more important one: Did my character grow in some way today? Did I acquire a little bit more skill in self-control and perseverance? The answer to both those questions was "Yes." So did I succeed? Yes.

Amazing. I had almost written off my day as a failure because my step forward seemed so small and insignificant. But it was a step—the first step in acquiring a skill that would benefit me for life.

Don't underestimate the power of achieving a small goal. Both of us were all-or-nothing people and originally looked down on setting small goals. They didn't seem challenging enough to us, so we never set any. Our goals were always big ones that had no guarantees and were much riskier. Because of this, our victories were also fewer and farther between. This was a huge mistake because we missed out on laying a foundation of successes.

We learned the best way to rack up success is one small step at a time. This is really important because success breeds success. You do this by setting a goal that is right at the end of your fingertips. Something small and attainable, but also something that is going to require you to take action doing something you haven't already done. Then, as you begin to experience success, you can, little by little, set bigger goals.

Now it is your turn to take a step. What is the frontier you need to conquer?

Lara: To become skillful, I need to take small steps. I do this when cleaning the house. I focus on one room at a time, starting with the least dirty room. Once that room becomes spick-and-span in a matter of minutes, it gives me enough motivation to tackle the next dirtiest room. Don't overwhelm yourself with trying to apply this entire book all at once. Pick out concepts you think will be easiest to apply first. As you get those down, begin tackling more challenging ones.

Chapter 10 Take-Home Messages

✓You reap what you sow.

✓Your success or lack of success is tied to your habits.

✓You break bad habits by creating new ones to take their places. Don't focus on the bad habit, instead focus on creating new ones.

✓Simply give it your best shot, and if your attempt fails, take note, make adjustments, and then try again.

✓The first step of temptation usually occurs in your mind with a suggestive thought.

✓Ask yourself: Is this the wisest choice?

✓Use procrastination to your advantage by "running out the clock" when tempted to eat things you know you shouldn't eat.

✓Your survival kit is your go-to when experiencing uncomfortable/negative feelings or when in a funk.

✓Perfectionism kills, but freedom gives life.

✓Tracking allows you to connect the dots so you can set yourself up for success.

✓Utilize the resources right at your fingertips.

✓Don't underestimate the power of taking a small step.

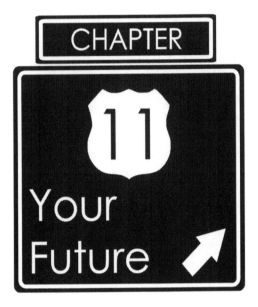

CHAPTER

11

Your Future

Mile Marker Peace

Lara

"We're home!" Hearing those words always reminds me of my Dad's voice from the front seat of the car as he pulled into our driveway after a long ride home from vacation. You would find my sisters and me sprawled all over one another with stiff necks and fatigue. Moans emerged from us as our parents would tell us to grab our bags and head into the house. And of course, just as our hands were full, we'd have to stand by the front door, exhausted, until someone *finally* found the house key. At last, we would spill into the house and run to sleep in our beds.

What does life look like for people after they get home from vacation? When you bump into other travelers as they are out exploring the world, you find them so happy and energetic. They are usually decked out in ski gear, sporting a suntan, or wearing a Hawaiian button-up shirt. Seeing them in this way always makes me wonder what their real lives are like. You know...when they get home and have to deal with the rawness of everyday living. That thought always piques my curiosity, because what you see isn't always what you get.

Well, friends, *we're home*. And the good news is the future doesn't have to be a complete mystery. We've visited so many different rest stops with you—the Land of Oz, the roadside fruit stands. We've reflected on our lives as we watched sunsets and climbed rocky cliffs together. Recording these stops on our journey has not only become a great way to self-reflect, but it gives you a clear outline of what makes you uniquely you.

You hold your map in the palm of your hand. This information is valuable, and it will always be here when you need it. You don't have to look into the future without a plan. This map already identifies what you want it to look like. And remember, if you ever get lost, the way back home is to *follow peace*.

We've mentioned countless times how your life is like no other, which is why diets don't work—they are unable to create a lifestyle that is tailored specifically for you. Only you can carry out that lifestyle. The cool thing is, now you have the goods. You know yourself on a deeper level after taking this journey, and you can continue to make adjustments until you find the happiness you've been yearning for.

Now that you are home and before we head our separate ways, we want to give you a clear picture of what following peace may look like in the future. We won't leave you wondering, especially since you've invested so much in our journey. We hope a glimpse of our lives will give you the encouragement you need to continue moving forward, despite the daily challenges you will experience when real life happens.

In some ways our lives will look the same, and in other ways we will be very different. That is the beauty of this journey! Every person will have a unique answer for what life looks like, but the destination will always be the same: a lifetime of peace.

Our "Aha" Moment

One of the most frequent questions people ask us is when did our initial "Aha" moment occur. Although we had our initial lightening in a bottle experience, described in the intro, it is hard to pinpoint the exact instant when we both began walking consistently in peace with food. We remember how we felt when our peace level began to go up, but it wasn't something that fell from the sky and zapped us. Our "Aha" moment is probably best identified by looking back from where we started this journey and what our level looks like today.

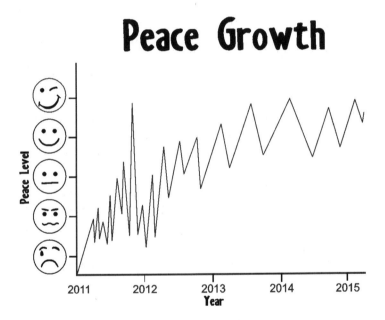

Back in our dieting days, we would have mostly bad days. The swings of our emotions were erratic and sometimes self-control was completely nonexistent. We would lose weight and be on a high, then cave to food and be down and depressed.

Once we began our journey and learned skills to find peace, our joy gradually improved after a rocky start. Over time, the bad days became less frequent, and the lows were further apart. We had more good days than bad, and our charted levels weren't as extreme. As time passed, the trend became a gradual improvement in our overall peace level. Even though we still have bad days, they aren't as bad as they used to be. Two things will happen over the course of your journey: your overall peace level will go up, and fewer big emotional swings will occur. Yea!

So, when does that "Aha" moment occur? Somewhere in the middle of our journey, we came to a significant realization: peace with food is a process. It is a process that we learned would take time and requires digging deep and really discovering how we thought about food. We learned that experiencing tranquility in any area of life is a never-ending commitment, but one worth fighting for.

Even when we understood this, we still had moments when we lacked patience. We're human, so it is completely natural to feel the need for instant gratification. But when we gave in to that temptation by cutting corners with a quick fix, we eventually found ourselves right back where we started. One small step, day by day, became our new motto, and thankfully it worked! This way of life is our new norm, one we never want to surrender.

We know the slow and steady approach isn't very enticing and may even be a disappointment for some of you. It took us a while to find peace, but it shouldn't take you nearly as long because we've already done the heavy lifting for you. We would be lying if we said we never had the urge to give up at one point or another, but in those moments, you have to ask yourself what is most important. Are you ready to make a life change and walk away from those extreme highs and lows we talked about? If so, you've got everything you need to make it happen. You've come this far. Don't stop now. You can do this!

Robynn's Life of Peace

Check-off lists. I'll admit I'm addicted to them. In fact, you will find them scattered around my house on pads of graph paper. On these pads are my goals, plans, dreams, and other random pieces of information I deem important enough to jot down. That's the achievement and visionary part of my personality. I get a great deal of satisfaction from setting goals and completing them. This is one of the ways I stay on track in my journey. Scribing my thoughts, goals, and dreams anchors my life and gives me clear direction and awareness.

The following is a snapshot of what following peace looks like at this stage in my life:

Good morning, World! My alarm typically goes off at 3:45 a.m. As odd as this may sound, I actually love waking up. The way I start off the morning frames my whole day. Many mornings I wake up before my alarm goes off because I'm excited to get out of bed and I have an inspiring reason to do so. Life wasn't always this way. I didn't always have a worthwhile purpose, and I can tell you that life was anything but exciting back then. But that has all changed.

I have heard people refer to your purpose as your life sentence. Here is mine: Be a blessing dispenser, helping others live their ultimate lives, lives of freedom, happiness, and fulfilled purpose.

As I begin my day, I whisper a prayer, *God help me be a blessing today.* The first hour of my day is reserved for reflection—reading the Bible, prayer, and listening to praise and worship music. Then I'm off and running. Literally! My exercise time, whether running or doing a workout DVD, usually includes listening to Joyce Meyer in the background. Remember, I thrive on accomplishment and this helps me maximize my time!

Proverbs 23:7 tells us "For as [a man] thinketh in his heart, so is he." I don't know of any activity that can change your mindset about yourself faster than exercise. At least that is true for me. In regard to the mental aspect of my journey, it ranks right up there for giving me the biggest bang for my buck.

Moving right along—time for more multitasking! To have the maximum amount of happiness in my life, I know that I need to look and feel my best. As I shower, step on the scale for a reality check, do my hair, and apply makeup, I listen to an inspirational teaching by John Maxwell or Willie George, my former pastor. This packs a big punch and makes me feel beautiful on the inside.

Wow, time flies! It's already 7:00 a.m. Time to wake my girls. We spend the next hour doing our morning routine—making our beds, practicing piano and violin, saying our Bible verses, eating breakfast, and getting our backpacks ready. If things go as planned, we are out the door by 8:00 a.m. But as we all know, things don't always go as planned. Since my life now focuses on following peace, I have learned to give my girls grace and, for the most part, just go with it. It is amazing how my journey has helped me see the big picture, which this morning is getting out the door at 8:10 a.m. versus 8:00 a.m. Now I spend more time investing in these two young girls and modeling a life of peace. I am not perfect in these endeavors, but I am far from where I was when I first started.

By 8:30 I am sitting down with a chocolate protein shake. Boy, do I enjoy my protein shakes. They keep me satisfied all morning and keep me on the right track eating-wise. I walk away from them feeling satisfied, a far cry from my past when I would eat way too many calories and end up with a feeling of GUILT! And you know what guilt leads to…an insane cycle of consuming even more calories!

The day rolls on, and I'm in my work mode doing what I love to do—writing, speaking, coaching, and studying. Lara and I work on projects. I study personal growth, look for opportunities to send an encouraging word to someone, and think, *Wow, does life get any better?* They say it's not work if you love what you're doing.

At 11:00 a.m., it's lunchtime, and the fact that I waited this long to eat shows how far I've come. I used to eat all my calories for the day at breakfast, causing me to either feel deprived the rest of the day or to overindulge. Either way it had a very detrimental effect on me. But not anymore. I now wait until lunch to eat a moderate meal. This sets me up for success the rest of the day. As a former grazer who would crash and burn mid-afternoon, I have now developed a habit of snacking on fruits and vegetables.

Afternoons are filled with more work, and then at 3:30, it's time to pick up kiddos! Once we are home, we spend the rest of our day doing homework, eating dinner (preferably a healthy one with a protein and vegetable), playtime, and bedtime routines—that include story time and prayer. By the time my girls are asleep, I'm ready to head to bed. As my head hits the pillow, I'm thankful. Thankful for my family and friends, thankful for my health, thankful for my many blessings and yes, thankful for peace with food. I am truly blessed.

Robynn: As far as my weight, I am currently at the top end of my optimal weight zone. I experience the greatest peace when I'm in this ten to fifteen pound zone. Vacations and holidays sometimes cause me to get outside of my zone, but I've learned how to get right back on by not panicking and hitting the reset button.

Lara's Life of Peace

Lara

It's 4:15 a.m. and the alarm goes off. The thought of hitting "snooze" crosses my mind, but a lot of work must be done before the kids wake up. I tiptoe out of the bedroom to avoid waking my husband and head to the kitchen to start the coffee. *If everything goes as planned I can get a devotion read before my day truly begins.*

I open my Bible. Just as I sit down to enjoy my first sip of caffeine, I hear a kid stirring. *Noooo!* I instantly freeze…so much so that I refuse to blink. The slightest movement could be all it takes to awaken my restless child. *Whew! I'm in the clear. Time for some good one-on-one God time. Lord knows I could use Him to sand my rough edges.*

Fast forward two hours, and the house is in full swing. The kids' hot chocolate is in the microwave, school papers need to be signed, "surprise" laundry needs to be started because our little one peed the bed last night. "Kids, what do you want for breakfast?" I ask. "Your shoes are on the wrong feet." The questions and commands become an endless clamor throughout the room.

By 8:30 a.m. I realize I haven't eaten breakfast, and I see my son's unfinished Pop-Tart on the counter. *Should I eat it as I tidy up the kitchen and head to the freezer for my homemade breakfast energy balls? Nope. Not going to waste my calories on that.* The leftover Pop-Tart goes into the trash.

I begin juggling a little book writing, cuddling, answering email, talking to Robynn, laundry, and debating on a time to get in some exercise. *Lara, if you don't exercise before noon, you'll be more likely to avoid it altogether.* I set the timer for thirty minutes, text a friend a picture of my messy house, and clean like a mad woman until my time is up. I wipe the sweat from my face and text my friend an "after" picture. *Exercise and clean house complete. Check.*

I walk past the mirror in the bathroom as I put the towels away. I remind myself I need to freshen up. *Even if I just pull my hair in a ponytail and apply some eyeliner, I know I will feel so much better the rest of the day. Wait. What is that? A new sunspot?!* I get friendly with the mirror and spend a few seconds getting lost in my frustration with my skin changes now that I'm getting older. *Hold on. I'm not going there. Some things in life you don't have much control over, and this is one of them.* I hear a child request my help. I quickly fix my hair and throw on some makeup. Back to work.

After trying to multi-task, I catch myself having a mental pep-talk so I don't "lose it" with my kids. I feel like I've had a constant tapping on my shoulder all afternoon. The phone keeps ringing, a kid needs me, the dryer hums, a negative thought bounces around in my head. *Fight the urge, Lara. Hold your composure. Lord, help me! Take a deep breath.*

I sit down and begin to work on the book. I hear my son in the other room repeatedly making rocket ship sounds. I stop typing and chuckle to myself. If my readers only knew what my writing conditions were like. *God, thank you for your humor.*

I think of an idea for the book, so I quickly jot down the following words on the back of my daughter's graded homework:

My human tendencies make me want to gravitate to the negative side of life. I have to deal with these feelings like everyone else, but having the "follow peace" reminder in my back pocket helps a great deal. When I feel like I am drowning in dirty dishes or junk mail, I have to stop and ask what is going to give me peace. In those moments I learn to be okay with whatever that answer is, even if the outcome doesn't look perfect.

The kids are loud and demanding because they are hungry. *Whoa. Is it lunchtime already?* After I get them fed, I prepare a salad: lettuce, chicken, cranberries, cherry tomatoes, cheddar cheese, buttery croutons, hard-boiled egg, and Honey Mustard Dressing. *Hold on, does this salad have as many calories as the leftover pizza? Oh well. I'm glad I had the patience to prepare it, because I enjoyed how it tasted and I don't feel sluggish. Not to mention, it has a lot of nutrition in there...somewhere...*

It's 1:30 p.m., and the kids are restless. *It's gonna be a long afternoon.* I try to play catch-up with whatever I didn't get finished in the morning. My son wants to play hide-and-seek, so when I'm "it," I purposely count slowly so I have time to swap out the clothes in the dryer. We get a little too noisy as we play and awake up my youngest from his nap. *Oops!*

The clock reads 3:00 p.m. The kids get fruit to tide them over until my daughter gets home from school. I head to the freezer to get my ½ cup of frozen trail mix and eat it while I drink a huge cup of ice water. I remember my time before my journey and give thanks for learning how to eat. Now, I won't be tempted to waste my calories on my daughter's after-school sweet treat later.

Once my daughter gets home, and the kids have their sweet treat, we tackle homework. As I tell my daughter her next spelling word, I find myself standing at the pantry door searching for food because I realized I didn't set out any meat for our evening meal. Like clockwork, my husband Doug calls to tell me what he plans to make for supper tonight. *I love that man.*

I begin daydreaming about how my husband has been a huge supporter in this venture. *I'm so lucky to be married to that guy. He read the book countless times for editing, gave me strength when I didn't have any left, and became as deeply rooted in this new approach to food as I was. In the past we would have talked each other into eating that last slice of lasagna or automatically including a dessert in our meal plan even if we were full. Nowadays you'll catch us reminding each other to stop eating if the food didn't meet our expectations. It's great to have that support and accountability, and hopefully it sets a good example for our kids. Thank goodness for this journey that has changed my life!*

"Mom. M-o-m! Are you daydreaming again?" my daughter asks.

The door opens. "Dad's home!" the kids shout as they race to the door. *I'm so glad he's home.*

Once dinner is made and we eat as a family, the kids run off to play until it's time for baths and storytelling. By the time the kids are snug in their beds and kisses are given, I head down the hallway to the kitchen. At this moment my holiday begins.

One frozen cookie dough ball from the freezer and one cold glass of milk. I carry them to the living room and set the stage. First things first: low lighting. I turn off the lamps and turn on my white Christmas lights. *People probably think I'm weird for having these up all year round. Oh well, I like them!* I put all of my favorite pillows on the couch, grab a quilt, and get snuggled in. *Shoot! I forgot the TV remote! Grrr!* I get up and do this all over again. *Ah, finally.* The house is quiet, the kids are sleeping, I get to hang out with my husband, and I can feel the tingling of my legs after a hard day of work. So…relaxing. I turn on the TV and take my first bite of cookie dough. Y-U-M.

I close my eyes for a brief second and savor every bite while soaking up these moments of "me" time. *I'm glad I passed up those stale cookies in the pantry earlier. This was so worth the wait.*

After some good laughs and reflecting on the day through conversations with Doug, my eyes get heavy. It's time for bed.

For the few brief moments before I drift off to sleep, I give thanks for my many blessings, peace with food being one of them. *Lord, thank you for helping me understand what peace really looks like. I couldn't have done this without You.*

Lara: One thing you won't find in my narrative is referring to the scale. Typically, you won't find a scale readily available in our house. I don't like to feel controlled by it. If I am making good eating choices and getting adequate exercise, then I am doing what brings me peace. I don't want a scale to be a hindrance to my progress by constantly lurking over my shoulder. As far as my current weight is concerned, I am within five pounds of the all-time low in my adult life. Even if I stay right where I am, I have complete satisfaction with it. It's not the number on the scale that will bring me happiness, it's what's in my heart. And thanks to peace with food, I'm there.

216 | PEACE WITH FOOD

Happily Ever After

We have always held to the hope, the belief, the conviction that
there is a better life, a better world, beyond the horizon.
~Franklin D. Roosevelt

Lara

One night, as I finished reading my daughter a bedtime story, she jumped into her top bunk and said, "I love happy endings!" I smiled. "Me, too," I agreed. "Me, too."

We've all witnessed a story of an overjoyed princess who rides off into the sunset with her prince. She can't stop smiling because she has finally found true bliss. We often think this type of fairytale ending is unattainable. Well, think again. Peace with food gives the same feeling of delight and happiness as a princess who's captured her dream—feelings that many never thought possible in this area of their life. For once, an outcome with weight loss and food that has a happy ending!

I know it may seem difficult to believe what I am saying, but let me assure you, the tools in this book will change your life forever. All you have to do is apply them. Like Cinderella, who was finally rid of her stepmother, think how great it would feel to no longer let some crazy diet or unachievable deadline torment you. I still have to pinch myself that I no longer have to live this way. I am the one in control of what I eat, and I don't have to feel guilty about this area of my life anymore.

You deserve to be that smitten princess or prince who gets to spend each day in peace. Like falling in love with your special person, you can fall in love with peace. Even though this new life has its ups and downs, with each day your love grows deeper and stronger. The more patient you are, the more love you'll experience.

So don't put your life on hold any longer. Let peace with food give you the life you've always wanted and dreamed of: a life of happily ever after.

Chapter 11 Take-Home Messages

✓If you ever get lost, the way back home is to *follow peace.*

✓ Over the course of your journey, your overall peace level will go up and fewer big emotional swings occur.

✓Peace with food is a process that requires digging deep and really discovering how you think about yourself, your body, your weight, exercise, and food.

✓You deserve a life full of happiness and peace.

Afterword

If you asked us what our most valuable resource was while working toward peace with food, we would say, "Having someone to share the journey." Being able to travel along with another person was the cherry on top, if you will.

Utilizing your posse makes the experience easier and more enjoyable and helps keep you focused on what you are working toward: peace (which will ultimately result in weight loss).

The reality is that even though we knew the end result would be peace, the human side of ourselves had moments when we got impatient with the results. We were often tempted to go for the quicker diet mentality because it is plastered everywhere in our society—the Internet, television, magazines, you name it. It was easy to question whether working this out—slow and steady—was really going to pay off. Luckily, we never shared these feelings of doubt at the same exact time. Being able to talk to one another always brought the doubtful one back on track. Yet another benefit to having a posse.

If at all possible, we encourage you to take this road trip through the book with someone else. If you can't think of anyone to share it with, that is okay too. Don't let that keep you from starting. This book is designed to help anyone, whether it is one person or an entire group. Again, you have to know yourself, so do whatever you feel is best for you!

Whether driving solo or with a group, we have included a *Posse Discussion Guide* to help facilitate your journey. You can decide how to break up the suggested discussions in order to accommodate the pace and time you want to devote to each. A blank notebook would also be helpful to journal your responses.

Gather your posse frequently. Share your thoughts on the discussion guide together. Have everyone read the assigned vignettes and answer the coordinating rest stop and journal questions before each meeting. This way you can use your time to discuss your findings and responses as a group.

Follow-up meetings would be beneficial in the months after your group discussions have concluded. This will serve as your accountability time to check in and share struggles and victories. Use this time to help one another by sharing your recent experiences in your walk in peace with food.

After brainstorming with your posse, make note of ways you can adjust what you are currently doing, and schedule follow-up conversations if you feel the extra support will be helpful.

No matter what you chose to do, there is no right or wrong way to work through this. The most important thing is to get started. So...let's begin!

Posse Discussion Guide

Life is better together! We believe it so much that we have created this *Posse Discussion Guide* to assist in sharing a life of peace with your posse.

The goal in having a posse is to pull together one or more individuals you can trust, be open with, and rely on during your peace with food journey. You can be as flexible as you like on how often, when, how, and where you meet. If meeting in person is too difficult, consider utilizing an online private forum to work through the guide. It may take a few weeks or even months before people begin opening up, but with every gathering, we think you will find yourself peeling back one layer of discovery at a time. The goal is to build camaraderie and increase your level of peace.

The following guide can be used to take you through the book. We suggest you read each chapter before going through the posse guide questions. Here are a few tips to help you understand our layout:

- Words in *italic* specify the vignettes within the chapter we are referencing.
- The **X** symbol signifies the rest stop(s) within that chapter. Those questions should already be filled out within your book.

If you are interested in leading a posse through this guide or want to dive even deeper on your own, you can purchase our *Leader's Discussion Guide*. It comes fully scripted and includes additional activities and reflection questions to do with a group or on your own. We also have a *Bible Study Posse Guide* along with the corresponding *Bible Study Leader's Guide*.

So grab your journal and your posse and begin embarking on this new and everlasting journey called *Peace with Food*.

Chapter ❶: Best Life Ever
1. In the vignette *Meet Lara & Robynn*, they each share their diary. Journal about your life experiences with your body image, food, weight, and exercise. What would "your diary" say?

2. After reflecting on what your life looks like now, what does your best life ever look like? Take a few moments to write down specifics regarding how this life would look and feel. Use the following list to help you in visualizing your best life ever. How would you like your life to look in these areas?

- Spiritual
- Personal
- Relational
- Physical
- Professional
- Financial
- Mental
- Social/Community Service
- Recreational

Chapter ❷: Diets Don't Work
1. Make a list of the diets you have tried in the past. Which ones were the most successful in the short run? The most difficult? Did any of them produce permanent results? Which ones gave you the most peace?

2. Below are some questions to think about. Whatever resonates with you, write your answers in your journal.
    A. In the vignette *Lacks a Permanent Solution*, Lara attempted the same diet as her sister and did not get identical results. Has this ever happened to you? How did it make you feel? What were the results because of it?
    B. *Too Much Focus on a Quick Fix* is about losing weight on a diet but not knowing what to do when you reach your goal. Do you find this to be true?
    C. *Results Are Not Typical*, unfortunately, is pretty common in the diet industry. The next time you wait in

the checkout line at your grocery store, count the number of magazines that make incredible claims about weight loss, and make note of the diet they are promoting. You may also want to see if the diet has a disclaimer at the bottom in small print that says, "Results not typical." Write in your journal the most outrageous claim so you can share it with your group the next time you meet.

D. Did reading *Success Is Based on Inflated Weight* parallel with your past experiences? What are your eating habits before you go on a diet? Do you pork out? Are you super focused? Stressed? Does overeating cause your weight to become inflated before your diet has even started?

3. *The Insane Cycle Dominates* vignette talks about our repetitive experiences with food, our body, and weight. Circle the following examples you can relate to, then add your own insane cycle habits in the blanks below.

- Thinking the only way to get back on track is to not eat for a few days.
- Feeling like a failure when unexpected events cause me to overeat.
- Stepping on the scale multiple times a day.
- Thinking that food will satisfy when I am in a funk or having a bad day.
- Not realizing my obsession with weight is stealing my enjoyment and quality of life.
- Allowing little slip-ups to turn into full-fledged mess-ups.
- Buying healthy foods I don't like but feel obligated to get, only to pitch them weeks later because they spoil in the fridge.
- _____
  _____
  _____

4. Look back to *The Blame is Put on Food* and fill in the blanks below:

You can _____ whatever you want,
as _____ as it brings you _____.

5. What do you think about the above statement? Do you agree? Disagree?

6. *Heavily Influenced by They* discusses the unknown group of people who tell you how to live. Jot down rules given by "They." Include rules in any area you can think of (parenting, relationships, finances, fashion, your appearance, etc.).

7. After reviewing *It's a One-Size-Fits-All Approach*, in your journal, make a list that includes preferences and "must haves" in your life when it comes to food, exercise, and body. If you need examples, refer to the ones Lara and Robynn give in the vignette.

8. ✗ Refer back to the rest stop in *It's a Lab Setting, Not the Real World*. What are your personal situations, circumstances, and idiosyncrasies in your life that diets didn't take into consideration, causing you to fail?

Chapter ❸: Peace with Food
1. Glance back to *Follow and Rate Your Peace*. What are your thoughts on the peace chart containing faces? How do you think using this peace chart might come in handy for you? Rate your current peace levels in the following areas using the peace chart:

- Appearance/Body:_____
- Weight:_____
- Exercise:_____
- Food:_____

2. *Build Your Character* talks about character traits. Rate yourself from a -5 all the way up to a + 5 next to each of the character traits. Once you are finished, review the areas you scored lower than others. Next, write the name of someone you know who is strong in the areas that you are limited. This will be a good reminder to utilize those individuals when you need help in those areas.

- Spiritual
- Personal
- Relational
- Physical
- Professional
- Financial
- Mental
- Social/Community Service
- Recreational

3. After thinking about the *Simplify Your Life* concept, in what ways have diets complicated your life?

4. ✗ Refer back to your rest stop in *Experiment to Find What Works*. What diet "rules" have you adapted to fit your lifestyle because they have proven to be successful for you?

5. *Find What Keeps You in the Game* emphasizes the importance of recognizing what actions will be required for you to continue your walk in peace with food. What makes you feel best about yourself? Who will help contribute to your success? What events do you need to plan ahead for so you can stay on track daily? Make a list of things that you feel are important in your success.

6. Read *Choose the Outcome of Your Life*. Do you believe you are powerful? Yes or no? Explain.

7. *Live Intentionally* encourages you to live life on purpose. List out ways you could be more intentional. Here are some areas to consider:

- Spiritual
- Personal
- Relational
- Physical
- Professional
- Financial
- Mental
- Social/Community Service
- Recreational

8. *Benefit from a Posse* discusses the advantages of having a posse. What benefits do you see in having a posse?

9. After reading the entire chapter, pick one of the following questions to answer:
   A. What are your initial thoughts regarding peace with food?
   B. If you could sum up peace with food in one sentence, what would it be?
   C. Imagine what your life looks like once you are living at peace with food. Make a list of words that describe what your life looks like and how you feel.

Chapter ❹: Body
1. After reading *You are Not Alone*, have you ever felt alone in your weight loss attempts? What advantage would you have in being courageous enough to share your feelings with a trusted Posse Partner?

2. In regards to *Embrace Your Imperfect Self*, what part(s) of your body do you wish looked different? What part(s) can you change? What part(s) can you not change? How can you become content in those areas that can't change?

3 *Obsessing for No Good Reason* discusses areas of our body that we obsess over but no one else thinks about. What do you feel most self-conscious about, and what causes this emotional angst?

4. ✘ Refer back to your rest stop in *Look and Feel Your Best*. What makes you look and feel the best?

Chapter ❺: Mind
1. In this chapter, Lara and Robynn talk about the importance of knowing yourself.
   A. How well do you feel like you know yourself?
   B. If you could list one area you would like to know better about yourself, what would it be?

2. After reading *Determine Your Value*, do you see yourself as a perfect 10? Why or why not? If your answer is "No," how might you act and think if you did believe you were a perfect "10"?

3. Now that you've read *Choose a Purposeful or Purposeless Life*, imagine the most purposeful life you think you could live. What would it look like?

4. ✗ Refer back to your rest stop in *Do What Successful People Do*. List your affirmations regarding peace with food and a healthy body.

5. Do you need to *Get Real with Yourself*? If so, what specifically about?

6. In the vignette *Reset*, what one or two habits in regard to peace with food would change the course of your life? How could you begin to develop that habit?

7. ✗ Refer back to your rest stop in *Reset*. How can you use resetting to your advantage when it comes to food, exercise, or your weight on the scale?

8. Can you relate to the *Pitch the All-or-Nothing Mindset* vignette? Which approach do you use in regard to your eating? Explain why you think you use this approach.

9. Read *Give Yourself Grace*. On a scale from one to ten (ten being high) rate the amount of grace you give yourself. Then rate the amount of grace you give others. How can you be kinder to yourself, as well as others? How do you think giving grace to yourself will affect your journey?

10. ✗ Refer back to your rest stop in *Assess the Influence of Your Relationships*. What is the culture of your relationships regarding food or self-image? Include events that negatively impact your feelings regarding food, eating, or your body.

11. Journal about at least two of the following questions:
   A. After reading *Choose Peace over Panic*, do you ever hit the panic button? If so, under what conditions? What do you think you would need to do to hit the peace button rather than the panic button?
   B. Do you have funk days? How often do they occur?
   C. Lara shares an example of a funk day in the vignette *Recognize an "Off" Day*. What does a funk day look like for you?
   D. Can you see the benefit to *Take Advantage of a Rainy Day*? How can you help remind yourself of this tool the next time you are in a funk?

12. ✗Refer back to your rest stop in *Find a Posse Partner*. What can you do/whom can you rely on to stay motivated?

13. After reading *Get Help from God*, can you relate to this vignette? Does faith play a role in your journey? Do you ever feel like you are trying to hammer in one nail at a time and wish you had a "nail gun"? Have you enlisted help from above?

Chapter ❻: Weight
1. After reading *Be Smart with the Scale*, how often do you step on the scale? How would you describe your relationship to the scale?

2. ✗Refer back to your rest stop in *Decide What You Really Want*. What is it that you really want regarding your body and your weight?

3. ✗Refer back to your rest stop in *Find Your Optimal Weight Zone*. At what weight do you feel physically and psychologically best? What weight range does your dietitian/physician recommend? At what weight does your body naturally find the best fit for the predetermined physical attributes you've been given—your physical makeup, frame, musculature and metabolism? What weight gives you peace?

4. ✗Refer back to your rest stop in *Budget Your Calories*. Are you having a difficult time getting to your optimal weight zone? If so,

where are you overspending? Jot down where you are going over budget in your eating.

5. *Invest in Peace* talks about the price you are going to pay to get to your goal weight range. What price are you willing to pay? What is your bottom dollar you are willing to invest?

Chapter ❼: Exercise
1. Have you ever thought exercise was the answer to all your weight-loss issues? If only you exercised more, you would be at your optimal weight? In *Exercise Won't Solve All Your Problems*, we read about the marathon myth. Isn't it crazy to think someone who could run that many miles could actually gain weight? Have you had a similar experience?

2. After reading *Use a Variety of Exercise Routines*, were there any ideas Robynn shared that sounded interesting to you? Do you agree with mixing up your routine throughout the year, or do you like sticking to the same regimen?

3. Lara talked about her experience with *Non-Traditional Exercise*. What are your thoughts about this? Are there some ways you could get some nontraditional exercise in throughout the day? Journal all the ways you can add nontraditional exercise into your day.

4. ✗ Refer back to your rest stop in *Find an Exercise That Will Motivate*. What physical activities keep you in the game? What are your exercise preferences?

Chapter ❽: Food (A)
1. Glance back at *Counting Calories on a Twinkie Diet*. In your journal, jot down the number of calories you think you consume on a typical day. Next, use an online simulator to get a ballpark idea of the amount of calories you should consume daily, based on your current weight and height. Compare this number with what you are currently consuming. Were you close? What did this exercise teach you?

2. ✖Refer back to your rest stop in *Give Yourself a Psychological Release*. When do you need to give yourself permission to just enjoy food and have a Psychological Release?

3. ✖Refer back to your rest stop in *Overindulging Doesn't Bring Peace*. What are your reasons for eating out of bounds? What caused you to eat out of bounds during your last attempt at a psychological release?

4. Now that you've read *Determine Guilt vs. False Guilt*, can you distinguish the difference between the two? Share an experience having true guilt and one in false guilt.

5. ✖Refer back to your rest stop in *Making Healthy Choices*. What are you already doing that promotes healthy eating? What is one way you can include a new healthy selection in your day?

Chapter ❾: Food (B)
1. ✖Refer back to your rest stop in *Enjoying Comfort Food*. What is your comfort food?

2. ✖Refer back to your rest stop in *Don't Waste Your Calories*. What foods could you eliminate that are a waste of calories?

3. ✖Refer back to your rest stop in *Mr. Right vs. Mr. Right-Now*. What is your "Mr. Right" when it comes to food? (Your favorite foods.) What is your "Mr. Right-Now" when it comes to food? (Foods you eat because they are easily accessible.)

4. The *Bite #1 vs. Bite #21* concept can really be an eye-opener. Have you ever compared how something tastes when you consider the first few bites compared to many bites later? The next time you are faced with eating a Mr. Right food, conduct a little experiment. Take note of how the first bite tastes. Then record your results in your journal. When did you find that the food began to diminish in giving you pleasure?

5. How well do you create situations that *Have Closure with Food*? Or is this a new concept for you? In your journal, list a couple of practical ways you can begin getting closure in eating. (Ex: cutting recipes in half, buying individual sizes)

6. Can you relate to Robynn's experience in *Creating Situations You Can Control*? Is there any food you feel powerless over? Could it be that you need to cut it down to a moderate portion and get rid of the option of having more?

7. ✗ Refer back to your rest stop in *Restaurants and Travel*. What are some strategies you can use to successfully eat in peace while you are eating out or traveling?

8. ✗ Refer back to your rest stop in *Embrace Special Occasions*. How can you eat during the holidays in a way that will bring your soul comfort, but also peace?

Chapter ⑩: Action
1. After reading the beginning of this chapter, in regard to your body and health, if you keep planting the seeds you are sowing, what are you going to reap? What about other areas of your life?

2. ✗ Refer back to your rest stop in *Substitute Bad Habits with Good Ones*. What bad habits can you break by creating new ones?

3. ✗ Refer back to your rest stop in *Overcome Temptation*. What trips you up? (Food, situations, people, emotions, and time of day.)

4. How can you *Let Wisdom Do the Heavy Lifting*?

5. ✗ Refer back to your rest stop in *Be Prepared for a Temptation*. What strategies will help you outlast the temptation wave?

6. In *Use Procrastination to Your Advantage*, think back to an experience in which you could have benefitted by running out the clock. What was it?

7. Do you think you could get momentum by using the *Rip It like a Band-Aid® and Build Momentum* approach?

8. ✘Refer back to your rest stop in *Prepare for a Bad Day*. What items are in your survival kit to get you through challenging times?

9. After reading *Document Your Progress,* do you feel there is any benefit in writing down your progress or thoughts during your journey? After extensive journaling through this discussion guide, do you feel that it has been helpful?

10. ✘Refer back to your rest stop in *Utilize Your Resources.* What resources can help you live at peace with food?

11. ✘Refer back to your rest stop at *Develop Skills for Success.* What tools do you need to help you become skillful at living at peace with food and your body?

12. In the vignette *Make a Plan and Start Today,* take a look at the list of questions in constructing a plan. Do you see any benefits to having a plan? How realistic do you think it is to construct a plan and follow it?

Chapter ⓫: Your Future
1. In light of *Mile Marker Peace* and *Our "Aha" Moment,* let's answer the following questions:
   A. Reflect on your progress compared to when you started your peace with food journey. How far have you come?
   B. Do you have any concerns about the future?
   C. In what ways can you and your group help one another to continue with your journey toward peace?

Where do you go from here? It's time to intentionally create a plan that is tailor-made for you! Visit www.peacewithfood.com to start today!

Optional Reading Schedules

The book is broken down into the following chapters:
Chapter 1: Best Life Ever
Chapter 2: Diets Don't Work
Chapter 3: Peace with Food
Chapter 4: Body
Chapter 5: Mind
Chapter 6: Weight
Chapter 7: Exercise
Chapter 8: Food (A)
Chapter 9: Food (B)
Chapter 10: Action
Chapter 11: Your Future

Option #1—11 Week Study Discussion
Cover one chapter a week, meeting 11 times total.

Option #2—25-Week Study Discussion
There are 25 rest stops total. Have the group work through the book, stopping at each rest stop and answering the coordinating question. Only discuss one rest stop per meeting, therefore some weeks may require more reading than others, since some chapters have several rest stops and other chapters have none.

Option #3—Find what works for you!
Take it week by week or month by month! Go at whatever speed you find helpful! For more ideas visit www.peacewithfood.com

Notes

RESULTS ARE NOT TYPICAL
1. "Dieting Does Not Work, Researchers Report." ScienceDaily. *ScienceDaily.* 05 Apr. 2007. Web. 25 Feb. 2013.

EMBRACE YOUR IMPERFECT SELF
2. Horn, Sam. *What's Holding You Back?: 30 Days to Having the Courage and Confidence to Do What You Want, Meet Who You Want, and Go Where You Want* (New York: St. Martin's Griffin, 2000.), 111.

FIND A POSSE PARTNER
3. Olson, Jeff. *The Slight Edge*, 8th Anniversary Edition. Austin: Greenleaf Book Group Press, 2005-2013, 58.

FIND YOUR OPTIMAL WEIGHT ZONE
4. *Centers for Disease Control and Prevention.* Centers for Disease Control and Prevention, 04 May 2011. Web. 21 Mar. 2013.

COUNTING CALORIES ON A TWINKIE DIET
5. Park, Madison. "Twinkie Diet Helps Nutrition Professor Lose 27 Pounds." *CNN.* Cable News Network, 08 Nov. 2010. Web. 21 Mar. 2013.

INDULGE WITHOUT SACRIFICING PEACE
6. Palmer, Layla. "Brownie Batter." Web log post. *The Lettered Cottage.* The Lettered Cottage, 1 Feb. 2013. Web. 26 Feb. 2013.

MAKE A PLAN AND START TODAY Stephen Covey
7. Covey, Stephen R. *The 7 Habits of Highly Effective People: Powerful Lessons in Personal Change.* New York: Fireside, 1989. Print.

About the Authors

Lara is an entrepreneur at heart. Little did she know when ending her teaching career in 2007 to become a stay-at-home mom that she would start a thriving business.

Born and raised on a farm in Kansas, Lara was thankful for the country lifestyle and made special childhood memories with her three sisters. Despite savoring her upbringing, she had dreams of moving to a big city. In college she met her husband, Doug, also a farm kid, and moved to St. Louis, MO, shortly after graduation. Life continued to go the direction she'd always dreamt about. A couple years later, to her surprise, they found themselves missing life on a farm. Today, you can find them back in Kansas living on her husband's childhood farm, where they couldn't be happier raising their three children, Leanne, Garrett, and Cade.

Although life went a different direction than anticipated, Lara loves raising her children in the same environment in which she grew up. During the busy farming seasons, she enjoys helping her husband when she can—taking him meals and visiting during his breaks, while their kids play in the dirt.

When she isn't caring for her children or enjoying time with her husband, you can find Lara working on some type of project, whether it be a home decor remodel, a new book, or pondering her latest dream.

It's a small town but a great big life. That's the way Robynn feels about the little Kansas town where she lives with her husband Scott, a surgeon, and their two daughters Sophia and Isabella.

Like Lara, Robynn grew up on a farm, and her experiences growing up have given her a great appreciation for the simple pleasures of life: driving by corn fields in the summer, watching her children chase fireflies on a hot summer night while listening to the cicadas sing, the nostalgia of fall and a high school football game, the first snowfall, and her husband's cooking and humor.

Robynn has always loved working with people and helping them become the people they were designed to be. She fulfilled this passion as a former high school science teacher and now as a wife, mom, speaker, author, and Peace Coach.

Robynn spends her time teaching junior high and high school kids how to find their purpose, teaching leadership, writing books, and speaking. She is a John Maxwell certified speaker, trainer, and coach; a Certified Human Behavior Consultant; and she loves to learn about personal and spiritual growth.

She hopes someday to pursue her dream hobby of renovating/building cottages, furnishing them, and then giving them away to veterans who have been wounded in combat.

Check out the Peace with Food Bible Study

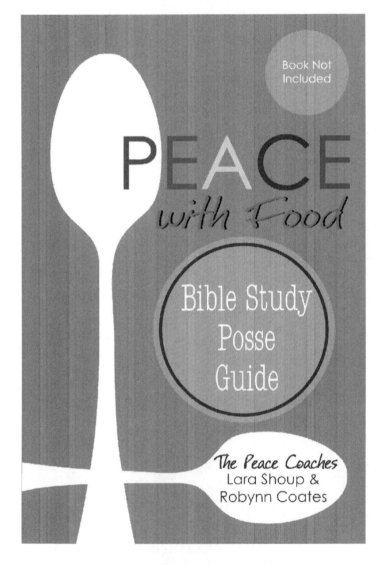

www.peacewithfood.com

Made in the USA
Lexington, KY
24 August 2015